A Practical Approach To
Saliva Control

by

Hilary Johnson, Dip.Sp.Th., M.A. (Ed.)

and

Amanda Scott, B.App.Sci.

Illustrations drawn under contract by Corwyn Zimbleman

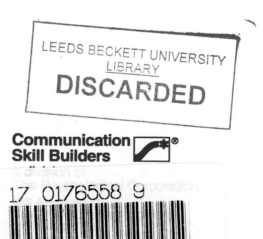
**Communication
Skill Builders**®

a division of
The Psychological Corporation

Reproducing Pages from This Book

As described below, some of the pages in this book may be reproduced for instructional or administrative use (not for resale). To protect your book, make a photocopy of each reproducible page. Then use that copy as a master for photocopying.

A Note of Caution

It is strongly recommended that health-care professionals wear surgical gloves when handling saliva in their treatment of clients with saliva or drooling disorders.

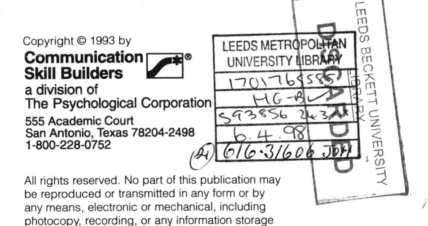
The Learning Curve Design is a registered trademark of The Psychological Corporation.

Printed in the United States of America

ISBN 0761678956

10 9 8 7 6

ABOUT THE AUTHORS

Hilary Johnson is a speech-language pathologist trained in England and now working in Australia. She has had a long-term interest in the area of severe communication impairment and, in particular, saliva control. In 1990 she completed a research thesis on the measurement of drooling. In 1992, she was awarded a Winston Churchill Fellowship to travel and investigate the available services for people with severe communication impairment in Europe and North America. Currently, she is working as the chief speech-language pathologist at the Spastic Society of Victoria in Melbourne, Australia. She is a member of the Saliva Control Clinic at the Royal Children's Hospital and a member of the Saliva Interest Group.

Amanda Scott is speech-language pathologist and Senior Clinician at Bethlehem Hospital in Melbourne, Australia. This hospital specializes in the care of adults with progressive neurological diseases such as multiple sclerosis and amyotrophic lateral sclerosis, conditions that have a high incidence of problems with salivation. She also has an interest in motor speech disorders and dysphagia and is undertaking research in this area. She is a member of the Saliva Interest Group.

CONTRIBUTING AUTHORS

Chris Bennett, M.B.B.S., F.R.A.C.S., is a plastic surgeon at Monash Medical Center, Melbourne, and in private practice. An original member of the Saliva Control Clinic at the Royal Children's Hospital in Melbourne, Mr. Bennett has had many years of experience in surgery to ameliorate problems associated with salivary function.

Libby Ferguson, B.App.Sci., is a speech-language pathologist at the Royal Children's Hospital in Melbourne, where she works mainly with young children who are developmentally disabled and infants who have eating difficulties. She attends the hospital's Saliva Control Clinic. Before beginning at the Royal Children's Hospital eight years ago, she was employed for many years at centers for children and young adults with intellectual disability.

Bronwen Jones, B.App.Sci., is presently a senior clinician in speech pathology at the Spastic Society of Victoria and conducts a small private practice. She received her degree from Lincoln Institute (LaTrobe University), Melbourne, and most of her career has focused on augmentative communication and working with people with severe and multiple disabilities. She has also worked in the Australian Outback in an educational setting and in an isolated country town in a general hospital. Since 1989 she has been Head of Department in a day-care center that runs programs for adults and preschool children who have severe and multiple disabilities, predominantly cerebral palsy. Working with clients to help them manage their saliva problems is an important part of her daily clinical role.

Susan Mathers, M.B., M.R.C.P., F.R.A.C.P., is a neurologist at Bethlehem Hospital and Monash Medical Center, Melbourne. Her main interests are the neurophysiological control of sphincter mechanisms and clinical issues in the management of patients with chronic progressive neurological disability.

Dinah Reddihough, M.B.B.S., Director of Child Development and Rehabilitation, is a senior pediatrician in the Department of Developmental Disabilities at Royal Children's Hospital, and chief instigator of the Saliva Control Clinic. She is also a member of the Saliva Interest Group.

Gloria Staios, B.App.Sci., is the chief speech-language pathologist at the Yooralla Society of Victoria, and has had a long association with children with severe disability. She is a member of the Saliva Interest Group.

Denise West, B.App.Sci., is a speech-language pathologist who trained in Melbourne, Victoria. She has worked in hospital settings and more recently at day-care centers, special schools, accommodation settings, and workshops for the physically and intellectually impaired. She has developed an interest in saliva control and oral-motor functions due to her work with children and adults with cerebral palsy who have requested assistance and programs to minimize their drooling. Ms. West has been involved in a research program that included trial use of the ortho-munchie on several adults. She has also worked with many clients in trial behavior modification programs, medication, surgery, and oral appliances in an attempt to reduce drooling.

CONTENTS

LIST OF FIGURES

LIST OF TABLES

PREFACE

In the early 1980s, a group of speech-language pathologists in Melbourne, Australia, commenced a saliva control interest group. In the course of our clinical and research studies, we came to realize the importance of the role of saliva and the problems often remaining with saliva after surgical interventions. Thus we changed our name to the Saliva Interest Group to reflect our broadening interest in the area. About this time, the Saliva Control Clinic was established at the Royal Children's Hospital in Melbourne. Since then a range of professionals working in the developmental and acquired disability areas have met and discussed their clinical observations and published findings, which form the basis of the chapters that follow.

Our aim is to introduce the topic of saliva and drooling to therapists, special educators, and caregivers. The book deals mainly with drooling, as this is a greater presenting problem in therapy services than the effect of a dry mouth. For the developmental population the current policies of deinstitutionalization and integration have introduced students with special needs into a wide range of school settings. A number of these students have an intellectual and/or physical disability that can result in an inability to control saliva adequately. It has been estimated that between 10 and 38 percent of children with cerebral palsy have a problem with drooling (Ekedahl and Hallen 1973; Makhani 1974; Van de Heyning, Marquet, and Creten 1980), as do 33 percent of people with a severe intellectual disability (Oreland, Heijbel, Jagell, and Persson 1989). Drooling often occurs in young infants without a disability but usually has disappeared by the time the child is two years old. For adults with acquired and progressive disorders there are no figures for the prevalence of saliva and drooling problems, but we know clinically that these people are frequently not given assistance in these areas.

The embarrassment and social isolation that accompanies drooling has often meant that both children and adults avoid certain activities and situations or endure negative community attitudes.

For those people who, for a number of reasons, are unable to effectively and regularly swallow their saliva, treatment has ranged from developing oral muscular control to the surgical excision of the saliva glands or ducts. These have often been applied from a "least intrusive to most invasive hierarchy"; from assisting with the development of oral sensorimotor control, to behavioral programs and orthodontic appliances, and finally to the more invasive medical and/or surgical intervention.

This range of intervention has involved speech-language pathologists, occupational therapists, physiotherapists, psychologists, dentists, doctors, and surgeons, depending on the courses of action prescribed. Unfortunately, rarely has a team approach been applied to the problem of drooling. This has resulted in a fragmented approach to both the assessment and treatment of the problem.

The following chapters present a team approach based on both theoretical and clinical expertise. Chapter 1 introduces the anatomy and physiology of saliva production. Chapter 2 outlines a method of dealing with saliva secretions for people with acquired and progressive disabilities. Also described are the important team members and an assessment procedure for children and adults (predominantly presenting with a developmental disability) with a saliva loss problem. Possible methods of measuring the drooling are also included. Chapter 3 explains a range of treatment possibilities. Finally, Chapter 4, which deals with compensatory strategies, identifies a number of ideas that can be incorporated into the program of a person for whom saliva control procedures may not have been fully successful. They are also ideas that can be used before any program of saliva control is formally instituted.

This book is not designed to be a cookbook of recipes. It offers a framework to assessment and measurement and outlines a range of interventions. A list of references for further reading is provided as well. The remediation of saliva loss is still incompletely understood. Only by listening closely to people with saliva control problems and their caregivers will we continue to refine and create treatment methods. We hope that people will use our reproducible assessment forms and respond with suggestions regarding additions that we need to make in any of the areas covered.

—*Saliva Interest Group, 1991*

Chapter 1 THE PRODUCTION OF SALIVA

Saliva has seven major functions:

1. It protects the teeth and gums and assists with oral hygiene.
2. It lubricates food to assist with chewing and prepares the food into a bolus for ease of swallowing.
3. It lubricates the tongue and lips during speech.
4. It facilitates taste.
5. It destroys micro-organisms and clears toxic substances.
6. It initiates carbohydrate digestion.
7. It regulates acidity in the esophagus.

Anatomy and Physiology of Saliva

The major salivary glands are the parotid, submandibular, and sublingual (see figure 1). The submandibular glands secrete 60 percent of the total saliva at rest and the parotid glands 25 percent, while the sublinguals and minor mucous glands provide the remaining saliva. The parotid glands secrete saliva through Stenson's ducts near the second maxillary molar tooth; the submandibular glands secrete saliva through Wharton's duct on either side of the frenulum of the tongue; and the sublingual glands secrete saliva through several ducts in the floor of the mouth. Each pair of glands produces different types of saliva. The parotids produce serous (thin and watery) secretions and are particularly important when eating and drinking. The submandibulars have both serous and mucous (more viscous) secretory cells but predominantly serous secretions. The sublinguals are also mixed but produce predominantly mucous secretions. Generally, more saliva is produced when people are awake, and there is strong evidence to support definite circadian rhythms. In fact, saliva production peaks in the midafternoon (Dawes and Ong 1973). It is also possible that we have circannual rhythms, but this has yet to be fully researched (Shannon 1966). Within these broad patterns of saliva production individuals have their own patterns of saliva production.

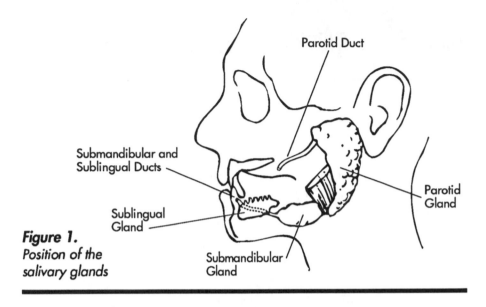

Figure 1.
Position of the salivary glands

Neurophysiological Aspects of Saliva Production

The complexity of the regulation of saliva production is still not fully understood. The salivary glands are regulated by the autonomic nervous system, which governs involuntary reactions.

The autonomic nervous system has two divisions: the sympathetic and the parasympathetic. The salivary glands thus have dual innervation. The parasympathetic division is more active on a regular daily basis and its influence leads to an increased flow of more watery saliva. The sympathetic division is more active during times of stress (fear, anger, etc.) and its activity results in more mucoid viscous saliva (hence the experience of a dry mouth when scared, or ropey saliva after hard physical activity). The variation in the saliva type (mucoid or serous) therefore occurs because the two autonomic divisions stimulate production of either more serous saliva (parasympathetic) or more mucoid saliva (sympathetic).

The parotid gland is innervated by branches of the glossopharyngeal nerve (IX cranial nerve). These branches originate in the inferior salivatory nucleus in the medulla and are parasympathetic. The submandibular and sublingual glands are innervated by branches of the facial nerve (VII cranial nerve), in particular the chorda tympani nerve. These are again parasympathetic and originate in the superior salivatory nucleus in the pons. The salivatory nuclei are not discrete structures but are contiguous. Sympathetic innervation to the salivary glands originates in the intermediolateral cell column of the first and second thoracic cord segments. These fibers synapse in the superior cervical sympathetic ganglion and travel to the glands via blood vessels (figure 2).

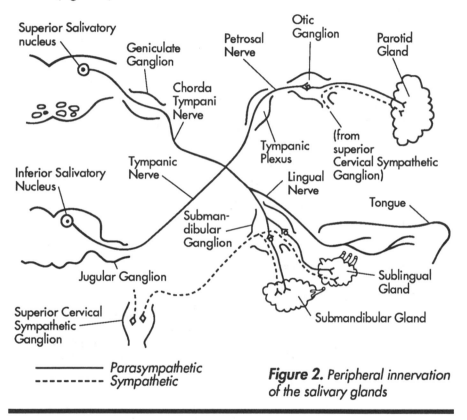

Figure 2. Peripheral innervation of the salivary glands

The cerebral cortex integrates the effects on saliva flow from both internal and external stimuli. There also appears to be an internal homeostatic mechanism that regulates saliva flow. Thus, if for some reason saliva flow is reduced (perhaps by surgical removal of a gland), there may be an increase in the flow of saliva from other glands to reinstate the homeostatic balance.

Researchers persist in attempting to establish a mean flow rate that is considered representative of normal in order that conditions such as hypersalivation (too much saliva) and xerostomia (a dry mouth) can be diagnosed. This rate is established by combining several results from different studies. Sreebny and Broich (1987) estimated unstimulated (resting) whole saliva at 0.3-0.5 ml/minute and stimulated saliva (by 2 percent citric acid solution) at 1.0-3.0 ml/minute.

Influencing Factors on Saliva Production

There are many factors influencing saliva production (figure 3) including gender, age, hydration, chewing, taste, sight of food, smoking, visualization, light, posture, mood/psychosis, disease/nerve damage, and medication.

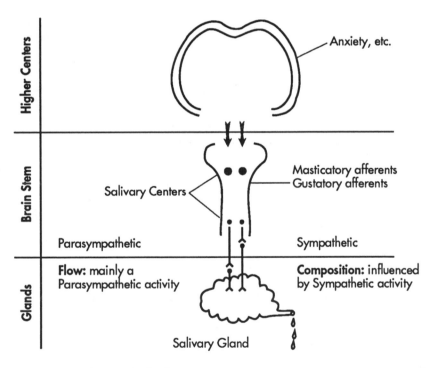

Figure 3. Neural control of salivary activity. Diagrammatic representation of afferent and efferent pathways that are involved in reflex salivary secretion under the coordinating control of salivary centers. These are in turn influenced by higher centers and, in this manner, anxiety, etc., may have effects on the reflex flow of saliva.

Gender

The effect of gender is not yet fully explained. In both the White (1975) and the Lagerlüf and Dawes (1984) studies, gender differences regarding whole mouth saliva were statistically nonsignificant. However, there was a trend that indicated males secreted more on each trial. A study by Andersson, Arviddson, Crossner, Holm, Mansson, and Grahnen (1974) demonstrated that stimulated whole saliva showed a significant gender difference, with girls having lower stimulated flow rates than boys. Crossner (1984) also stated that boys have consistently higher flow rates than girls. The effect of gender was significant only in the studies using a large number of students. Crossner (1984) also stated that gland size is the best predictor of saliva secretions. Although opinion is still divided, there are a number of studies that indicate it is possible that gender contributes to differences in the rate of saliva flow.

Age

Andersson et al. (1974) found that both the mean rate of unstimulated and stimulated whole salivary flow has been shown to increase up to the age of 15 years. Unstimulated saliva in boys in the 13-year-old age group showed a significantly higher flow rate than girls in a similar age grouping. With the younger subjects, the lower flow rates may well have reflected inadvertent swallowing of the saliva during the collection period. The reason for the increase in saliva flow could again be linked to gland size. As the children increased in age, gland size would also increase and more saliva would be produced.

Lourie's (1943) results did not agree with Andersson et al. (1974), with the mean rate of saliva flow decreasing rapidly from three to six years and less rapidly to fourteen years. The limited number of subjects in each age group (minimum of four and maximum of eight) cautions the extrapolation of these results. The age of the article may indicate less sophisticated techniques that are not considered as reliable as more modern collection devices.

Researchers also speculate that hormones contribute to rhythmic variations in saliva flow rates. (Dawes 1972; Palmai and Blackwell 1965). This is particularly important in females at or above the age of menstruation. It may be that menstruation affects the rate of saliva flow. Puskulian (1972) studied the stimulated flow in a small study that showed a lower flow rate at ovulation than during other parts of the menstrual cycle. Postmenopausal women have also been shown to have a saliva flow rate of 25 percent less than their premenopausal counterparts (Baum 1981).

There is also controversy among researchers in the literature on saliva production in the aged population. Frequently it is stated that saliva production decreases. When the effects of age, dentition, medication, and disease are taken into account, however, there appears to be a flow rate very similar to that of younger people, especially in stimulated saliva. The effects of losing teeth in the aged does pose a problem with eating, and Idowu, Grase, and Handleman (1986) state that masticatory function significantly declines with age. This in itself could affect the flow of saliva.

Hydration

The assumption that thirst comes from having a dry mouth is true for some people but not for all. Although recent research is scarce in this area, Holmes (1964) determined that reducing body water content did reduce the unstimulated saliva flow, and correlated dehydration with a lessened saliva flow in proportion to the degree of water lost. However, stimulated saliva after both mechanical and gustatory influence did not show any effects of dehydration. Since the range of what might be termed "normal saliva flow" is currently wide, general agreement about what is "dry" is important. If a person had a relatively high normal flow rate, a reduction in saliva flow might cause the individual to experience a dry mouth, while saliva flow measures could be within normal limits. Also the viscosity of the saliva may be an important factor in the feeling of dryness. Absence of thick mucousy saliva can lead to a feeling of dryness in the mouth even when saliva flow is within "normal" limits (Sreebny and Broich 1987).

Chewing

There is general acceptance that chewing increases whole saliva flow (Navazesh and Christensen 1982; White 1975). Hector (1985) recorded the saliva flow of eight subjects as they chewed a cereal chosen for its qualities of dryness, hardness, brittleness, and lack of taste. Anesthesia was applied to the periodontal ligament during trials. A reduction in the saliva flow from the parotid was noted during anesthesia. This experiment demonstrated the contribution of the periodontal receptors to saliva flow. Jensen Kjeilen, Brodin, Aarss, and Berg (1987) showed that salivation increased with both frequency and force of chewing, which stimulated the periodontal mechanoreceptor. Their finding reinforced the major role of the mechanoreceptors in the parotid response to chewing. Where there is poor periodontal stimulation (perhaps with ill-fitting dentures or soft food) a lesser amount of saliva might be produced. These conditions would be most frequently found in the elderly population, in institutionalized settings, or among students with oral motor disabilities.

Taste

The study by Jensen Kjeilen et al. (1987) also examined chewing with regard to the influence of taste. Their results showed that salivation increased with both frequency and force of chewing but that the citric acid produced greater dose-dependent salivary increases than the chewing. Watnabe and Dawes (1988) also examined the influence of tasting and chewing on the flow rate of whole saliva with three foods: rhubarb pie, boiled rice, and raw carrot. The effects of taste elicited salivary flow rates that ranged from 73 percent to 87 percent of those elicited by chewing.

Combined Influences of Taste and Chewing

A study by Muniz, Maresca, Tumilasci, and Perec (1983) studied the response of parotid saliva to change in diet among 66 healthy boys who lived in a children's home. The main emphasis of the study was to look at salivary component changes for developing a nutritious and caries-reducing diet. The diet was based on animal protein, fresh fruits, and vegetables, and had a 24 percent overall higher caloric value than the previous diet. There was a 40 percent reduction in carbohydrates and an increase in fat. After 45 days on the diet, the response of the parotid to stimulation was significantly increased, by 40 percent when compared to pre-test measures.

Smoking

In general, it is agreed that smoking increases the flow of saliva (Macgreggor 1988; Pangborn and Sharon 1971). The overall flow rate could be double that before or after smoking.

Sight of Food

The sight of food is commonly thought to produce saliva—hence the phrase, "mouth-watering." However, this is not fully borne out in the research. Few studies (Birnbaum, Steiner, Karmell, and Islar 1974; Christensen and Navazesh 1984; Wooley and Wooley 1974) have looked at the effects of the presence of certain foods on anticipatory saliva flow. The results varied from no significant difference to one related only to certain foods, such as pizza and lemon slices.

Visualization

Using imagery to increase or decrease salivary flow rates has been researched by Shannon and Chauncey (1969), White (1978) and Wooley and Wooley (1974). The result from the parotid saliva study (Shannon and Chauncey 1969) suggested that visualization had no effect on salivation while the studies on whole saliva demonstrated an effect.

It appears that vivid imaging abilities may assist in controlling the saliva flow. This technique to reduce saliva flow may not be useful in the treatment of people with an intellectual or cognitive disability.

Mood/Psychosis

The awareness of emotional effect on saliva was made use of long ago in the "Indian Rice Test": If suspects in a crime were unable to swallow rice because of lack of saliva, they were assumed to be afraid of detection, and therefore to be guilty (Burgen and Emmelin 1961). A considerable amount of interest has been shown in studying the flow rate of saliva in relation to both depressive illness and emotional state. Numerous researchers (Busfield, Weschler, and Barnum 1961; Bolwig and Rafaelson 1972; Palmai and Blackwell 1965; Peck 1959) have studied flow rates in the area of the psychotic state. The results were similar in that a clinically depressive state reduced the saliva flow. Once the person had recovered, the flow went back to normal.

Stress and anxiety have also been proven to produce a reduced parotid saliva flow. Bogdonoff, Bogdonoff, and Wolfe (1961) compared personality types with the effect of a stressful activity (the approach of the dentist drill).

The subjects were assigned to groups A (aggressive) and B (defensive) after extensive questioning. The results indicated an increase in parotid saliva flow for group A and a decrease in parotid saliva flow for group B that were statistically significant in both groups. In one subject there was no change in saliva production. He perceived the stay in the dental chair as restful and away from the stresses of work. The results of this study suggested that those people rated as more aggressive were more likely to increase their saliva flow in an anxiety-provoking situation, while those whose patterns were more defensive were more likely to exhibit decreased saliva flow.

There have been few studies of the relationship between salivary variables and normal personality traits. Costa, Chauncey, Rose, and Kapur (1980) measured the parotid saliva flow rate of physically healthy men who were rated on the 1962 Cattell Sixteen Personality Factor questionnaire and a modified Eysenck Personality Inventory. These results were compared with the effect of being in an anxiety-provoking situation. It should be noted that the anxiety-provoking situation was unlike the stress situations described in the paper by Bogdonoff et al. (1961). Costa et al. (1980) referred to a broad and enduring rate of emotional instability rather than a specific state of emotional arousal. The hypothesis of Corcoran (1964) and Eysenck and Eysenck (1967) that the stimulated flow rate was higher in introverts was confirmed. However, Ramsay (1969), who closely duplicated the work of Eysenck and Eysenck (1967), was not able to find significant differences but did note that introverts on the average gave consistently larger flow rate responses than extroverts to gustatory stimuli. The results from the Bogdonoff et al. (1961) and Costa et al. (1980) studies are contradictory. However, as different personality measures and a different definition of stress were applied, different results can be expected.

Light

A study by Shannon, Feller, and Suddick (1971) stated that light influences the flow of parotid saliva, which reinforced the findings of other works by Barylko-Pikielna, Pangborn, and Shannon (1968) and Pangborn and Sharon (1971). Here, when blindfolds were used, the flow rate of saliva decreased markedly. It might well be that light provides the principal stimulus for this basal and continuous rate of resting secretion by the human parotid gland. It may also contribute to the reasons why saliva flow reduces during sleep. The effects of light, however, have been investigated only on the parotid gland and not on whole saliva.

Posture

Shannon (1972) reported the overall position of his subjects affected salivary flow rates. While standing they had higher flow rates and while lying they had lower flow rates than seated subjects. As little research has been completed in this area, Shannon's results remain to be confirmed.

Disease and Nerve Damage

Disease that affects the salivary glands has been shown to have an effect on the flow. Examples of these are Sjogren's disease, Bell's palsy, tumors on the salivary nuclei, and damage to the vagus nerve or chorda tympani. A reduced flow of saliva often results in a disordered swallow (Fox, Ven, Sonies, Weiffenbach, and Baum 1985; Hughes, Baum, Fox, Marmary, Yeh, and Sonies 1987).

It has also been suggested that gum disease will increase the amount of saliva in the mouth due to an increase of fluid from irritation of the mucous membranes of the mouth; this is common also among people with oral-motor disabilities.

Medication

There are more than 400 drugs that have been cited as producing a dry mouth (Sreebny and Schwartz 1986). Some of these include anorectic drugs, anticholinergics, antidepressants, antipsychotics, diuretics, sedatives and hypnotics, antihistamines, antiparkinsonians, and antihypertensives. Kapila, Dodds, Helm, and Hogan (1984) reported briefly on the use of both cholinergic (increase salivation) and anticholinergic (decrease salivation) drugs. Subcutaneous cholinergic stimulation on six subjects elicited a sixfold increase in saliva over the unstimulated saliva rate. The application of an intravenous anticholinergic on the same six subjects almost abolished salivation. (For further information, see the section Medications Used in the Control of Oro-Pharyngeal Secretions, page 61).

Some of the drugs used to control epilepsy may also increase salivation. We produce approximately one to one-and-a-half liters a day of saliva.

The Different Consistencies of Saliva

Two consistencies of saliva are produced in careful balance. These are serous (or watery) saliva and mucoid (thicker mucous) saliva. Each has its own role in swallowing and in the maintenance of healthy mucous membranes, dentition, and the sense of taste.

When evaluating a possible problem of salivation, it is necessary to consider whether the saliva appears excessive or scant, whether it is watery or ropy, and whether the problem is confined to the mouth or throat or both regions are involved.

1. *Serous (or watery) saliva* is produced primarily by the parotid glands. Its production is stimulated by chewing action. The saliva is secreted directly in the region of the second molars where it is mixed with any food being chewed. This enables food to be mixed with saliva and the formation of a swallowable bolus. Serous saliva is important for the formation of a bolus orally and the lubrication necessary for the bolus to pass easily down the throat.

   The presence of serous saliva combined with reduced lip closure and tongue movement leads to drooling and what appears to be an excessive amount of saliva. It is difficult to ascertain whether there is excessive production of saliva because the problem may be caused by a reduced ability to swallow and/or to control the saliva within the mouth. The problem may worsen around meal-times, when food has to be chewed.

2. *Mucoid saliva* is produced by the sublingual and submandibular glands; mucus is also secreted by minor glands in the mucous membrane of the mouth and pharynx. Mucoid saliva has a thicker consistency than serous saliva because it has a higher percentage of protein. The mucoid saliva provides a protective, lubricating film over the surfaces of the mouth and pharynx and is also mixed with food in the mouth while it is being chewed and prepared to be swallowed.

   An excessive amount of mucoid saliva may have several underlying causes. It may occur when there is a reduction in spontaneous swallowing that leads to secretions collecting in mouth and throat. Jaw weakness may also be a contributing factor because a reduction in chewing leads to less secretion of serous saliva, thus leaving mucoid secretions in the mouth and/or pharynx. This problem may be increased if the individual mouth-breathes, which causes the secretions to dry and become thicker. Dehydration associated with reduced fluid intake will also contribute to the problem.

   The presence of ropy or stringy saliva can impair normal swallowing as it contributes to web-like formations of secretions in the mouth, or more usually in the throat, which collect food during swallowing and retard its progress. Tenacious secretions also require greater muscular strength to be moved during swallowing. More seriously, they can cause obstruction of the airway.

Secretions in the throat may originate in the lungs and may collect in the larynx and pharynx if the individual's cough is too weak to clear the airway adequately. They may also be produced within the larynx and lungs if the individual is aspirating small amounts of food while swallowing. Aspirated material is irritating and mucous is produced in response to its presence.

Insufficient Saliva

Dry mouth, or *xerostomia,* is a significant reduction in the amount of saliva. This problem occurs in a condition called Sjorgen's syndrome, which is associated with rheumatoid arthritis. It also appears after oral irradiation for the treatment of cancer, as a side effect of certain medications such as antidepressants or antihistamines, when there is excessive mouth-breathing, and in response to dehydration. There are more than 600 medications that may cause a dry mouth. The aged populace is particularly at risk for having xerostomia.

Dryness of the mucous membranes of the mouth and throat can lead to problems with swallowing because the smooth movement of the bolus depends on adequate lubrication. This condition may also compromise the health of the oral and pharyngeal mucosa and the teeth.

Now that we have covered the basic mechanics of saliva production and neurophysiological influences upon the process, we can move on to a consideration of assessment and measurement techniques regarding saliva and drooling.

Chapter 2 ASSESSMENT AND MEASUREMENT

The assessment of saliva secretions and the assessment of drooling sometimes necessitate different approaches. Generally, problems with saliva consistencies occur in people who have acquired and/or have progressive disabilities. These people may or may not have a drooling problem. (The assessment of this area is covered under Assessment of Secretions, below.) Drooling in the developmental area—for example, people with cerebral palsy and/or intellectual disability, less commonly involves problems with saliva consistency (unless the condition commences after surgical intervention for drooling). The assessment and measurement strategies suggested for the developmental population appear under Assessment of Drooling, page 15. Treatment of both conditions requires a team approach, although the evaluation may have been completed predominantly by one person (usually a speech-language pathologist).

Assessment of Secretions

The first step in dealing with a salivary problem is to adequately investigate and describe the nature of the problem.

Asking the individual with a salivary problem or, if appropriate, the caregiver, to fill in an oral secretion assessment form is a good place to start (see Assessment Forms section, pages 22-30). This provides information about the presence, consistency, amount, and timing of secretions. This information can form the basis for management decisions. The measurements are spaced at intervals during the day, and are taken before and after food or drink so that the effects of these can be noted. In some cases it may be useful to monitor what food and fluid is taken and if there is something in particular that causes an increase in the amount of saliva or changes its consistency.

Assessment is subjective and the qualifications of "excessive" and "very excessive" require discussion with the person filling in the form. The clinician needs to observe the problem and gain an idea of how it is perceived by the measurer.

When base measures have been taken, the treating clinician, in consultation with the team, can make decisions about whether drying or thinning saliva is the best course. After the person with the salivary problem has been stabilized on a specific medication, a re-evaluation of the salivary problem will assist in determining the effectiveness of the medication. Clinical experience has shown that there is a tendency for the mouth to be dry in the morning and for the amount of secretions to increase during the day, especially after meals. The drooling problem usually peaks in late afternoon. This is in line with the Dawes and Ong (1973) findings regarding circadian rhythms.

The remediation of drooling can involve many people. Their roles are outlined in this section on the team approach.

Team Approach

Dentist. A regular dentist can fully assess the state of the teeth and gums. A dental hygienist may advise on the best way to keep the mouth clean. Where major work is needed to re-align the jaw, an orthodontist may be involved. A prosthodontist may be the professional who advises on prostheses. A dental technician may also be used to adapt prostheses for the mouth.

Doctor. A doctor/general practitioner may be the first point of referral for a drooling problem. This person will probably make a referral to a specialist who could be a pediatrician, an otolaryngologist, or a speech-language pathologist.

Occupational Therapist. An occupational therapist may be involved in intervention and assessment. Again, check that the person is experienced in the area of drooling and will be able to help with a detailed eating and drinking assessment.

Pediatrician. This is an M.D. specialist for children. This person may provide treatment but will also make referrals to other appropriate sources.

Physiotherapist. This person will probably be involved with seating modifications where a physical disability is associated with the drooling. The physiotherapist may also be involved with biofeedback as a treatment intervention.

Psychologist. Behavioral psychologists are often helpful in devising programs to decrease unwanted behavior. They may also help you structure a program to maximize the person's learning ability.

Neurologist. This person has a detailed knowledge of the nervous system and is a specialized physician; the neurologist is particularly involved in the prescription of medication.

Speech-Language Pathologist. A speech-language pathologist (SLP) is an expert practitioner in the oral-motor area and is involved in assessment and therapeutic management. The SLP will be involved with a detailed eating and drinking assessment.

Surgeon. This person will be able to perform any necessary surgery. However, all surgeons have areas of expertise (for example, head and neck, plastics, etc.). Before surgery is performed for drooling, check that the surgeon is experienced in this area. Usually the surgeons involved are otolaryngologists or plastic surgeons.

Alternative Therapists. There are many types of "therapists" who may claim to cure drooling. Some of these include hypnotherapists, acupuncturists, shiatsu therapists, and chiropractors. They may be of some help but will probably not provide a team approach and may have limited medical knowledge.

Assessment of Drooling

Drooling or *dribbling, saliva loss,* and *poor saliva control* are all terms that conjure up a fairly negative picture. We think of these conditions as a temporary stage in infancy that will disappear as a child grows up. Unfortunately, this doesn't always happen and the child enters school with a wet chin, sometimes chapped skin, and often an unpleasant odor. No one really knows quite why some children drool, but it is rarely because they produce too much saliva. Drooling can also occur after traumatic surgery, brain injury, or during a progressive illness where the inability to control saliva may be caused by a neurological deficit.

One of the major ways in which we channel saliva down our throats is by swallowing. We swallow more than 1,000 times a day. Swallowing is more frequent during the day than at night, when the flow of saliva almost ceases. A recent publication (Sochaniwskyj, Koheil, Bablich, Milner, and Kenny 1986) suggests that people with cerebral palsy swallow at 75 percent of the rate of the able-bodied population. Thus infrequent swallowing might lead to the pooling of saliva in the mouth and eventual spillage, which is what we know as drooling.

Where a drooling problem exists, there are a number of people who can help in exploring treatment options and fully evaluating the problem. A central figure in this process is often the speech-language pathologist. First, an evaluation is carried out.

How to Assess the Drooling

The two Assessment Forms, "Saliva Control Assessment" (page 22) and "Observation of Saliva Control Checklist" (page 25), are presented as guides and should be filled in with as much detail as possible. If the person who drools is unable to complete the form, it is best completed by familiar people (for example, teacher, partner, parent). The assessment has been devised to lead into appropriate methods of treatment. (See case study examples for decision making, pages 19-20.)

Using the Saliva Control Assessment Form

When interpreting the saliva control assessment results, please read the following.

Cause of Drooling

Sometimes a cause can be found for the drooling; it may be specific brain damage after an accident or illness, or the introduction of a medication. Sometimes the oral sensorimotor mechanisms are slow to develop. It is often useful to investigate any changes in the severity of the drooling over time before implementing treatment procedures.

Head Position

A head-down position often results in saliva pouring out of the mouth. If the answers to Questions 2 and 3 suggest the person who drools has a problem with head control, it might be necessary to involve a physiotherapist for advice. He or she can give suggestions that may assist in the development of head control. If the person can hold his or her head up but continually drops the head some behavior management advice may be useful (which is covered in the section entitled Behavior Management, page 44). Environmental modifications may also be necessary (see Compensatory Strategies, page 71).

Oral-Motor Abilities

Questions 4 and 5 probe the person's ability to easily hold the lips together. If the mouth is open all the time, it may be that the person breathes through the mouth and needs to keep it open. It is possible to mouth-breathe without drooling (15 percent of the population do it). However, if this is the main cause of the drooling, see the sections Appliances (page 56), Behavior Management (page 44), and Oral-Facial Facilitation (page 32).

In the case of the person who finds it impossible to bring the lips together see Behavior Management (page 44), Medications Used in the Control of Oro-Pharyngeal Secretions (page 61), and Surgical Management of Drooling (page 66).

Questions 6-10 investigate the ability of the person to eat and drink. Where there is any difficulty, a full eating assessment should be carried out to investigate whether improved eating skills can be developed. See the section Eating and Drinking Skills (page 31).

Questions 11 and 12 investigate the person's sensory feedback. If the person cannot feel the saliva on the lips, it will be very difficult to control. Remember the time you lost sensation around your mouth after you had anesthesia at the dentist? You probably held a handkerchief to your mouth and dabbed furiously. Imagine having to do that all day. Where sensory loss is around the outside of the mouth, see these sections for ideas: Behavior Management (page 44), Oral-Facial Facilitation (page 32), and Appliances (page 56).

If the person has a strong reaction to various foods and drinks, an eating assessment is necessary. It may also contraindicate the fitting of certain oral prostheses.

Swallowing

Questions 13 and 14 relate to the swallowing process. It is important to watch the person (look for the larynx moving up and down in the neck) and count the number of swallows occurring. It may be that the person can swallow with no difficulty (as seen when eating) but rarely swallows spontaneously. If you are not sure whether the person is swallowing, place a stethoscope beside the larynx and listen for a swallowing noise (a double click). In a young child, a swallow can sometimes be stimulated by a puff of air on the face. If you do see a swallow, look for what the person does with the lips and the tongue. This will help you answer Question 14. Sometimes the person needs to be taught to swallow (see Behavior Management, page 44, and Appliances, page 56). Sometimes the person is not cognitively able to understand the process of swallowing (see Medications Used in the Control of Oro-Pharyngeal Secretions, page 61, and The Surgical Management of Drooling, page 66).

General Health

Questions 15-17 probe the health of the person. Where general health is poor it may be necessary to perform an eating assessment for specialist and nutritional advice. Drooling can increase when a person is sick, and the improvement of health must commence before drooling treatment starts. Frequent colds, asthma, and allergies may indicate that the person mouth-breathes. It may be necessary to refer the person to an ear, nose, and throat specialist or some other type of medical specialist for further assessment (see Team Approach, page 14).

Regular medications may also affect the health status. Some medications for epilepsy can increase drooling; the name and dosage of the medication should be noted.

Self-Stimulatory Behaviors

Question 18 relates to external behaviors that might increase the drooling, such as hand sucking. It is important to ascertain whether the drooling is due to the mouthing of objects or is actually drooling. In order to do this, it is necessary to observe the person when nothing is in his or her mouth. Some people may need to be physically restrained in order to keep the mouth free of objects. Others may need a range of different opportunities to practice exploring with their mouths (see Eating and Drinking Skills, page 31).

Where the drooling is predominantly due to external behaviors see a psychologist and read the section on Behavior Management (page 44).

Dental Health

Question 19 requires a full dental assessment, which is helpful in determining whether poor dental health may be contributing to the drooling (spongy gums often produce more saliva). A dentist can contribute greatly to the maintenance of good dental health. The assessment will also comment on the state of the dentition and the occlusion (bite). Where there is a large space between the front teeth on the upper and lower jaw it is important to know whether orthodontics will be able to correct the malocclusion.

Observation of Saliva Control

This form supplies a qualitative approach to the severity of the problem and can be completed before and after treatment. The questions mainly require a simple yes/no answer. This information is particularly useful in cases where the person doing the evaluation does not perform the treatment (as often happens with surgery). This information can be summarized when referring a patient for further investigation or treatment. (see Observation of Saliva Control Checklist, page 25). Two case studies follow that provide examples of how the Assessment Form can be used.

Examples of Problem Solving Using the Assessment Form _____

Case Study 1: Brendan, aged four, has a moderate intellectual disability and presents with a saliva control problem. Brendan:
- can keep lips together (Question 5)
- is unable to suck through a regular straw (Question 6)
- is unable to lick food from lips (Question 7)
- is chewing only up and down (Question 9)
- is usually healthy and is not on medication (Questions 15, 17)
- has good occlusion according to dental report (Question 19)

Age and eating difficulties indicated that intervention for Brendan's eating problems should be the first place to start.

Case Study 2: Kiara, a 15-year-old with multiple and severe disabilities, presents with a severe saliva control problem. The parents reported that Kiara had extensive intervention to improve her eating skills. She has no functional speech or formal communication system. Kiara:
- has always drooled (Question 1)
- is limited in her ability to keep her head up (Question 2)
- has her mouth habitually open (Question 4)
- tends to suck her mashed food (Questions 9, 10)

- is on medication for epilepsy (Question 17)
- has a moderate malocclusion that the dentist concluded would not improve (Question 19)

Here, because of her age and inability to control her saliva physically or intellectually, Kiara would not be able to take an active part in intervention. Surgery was suggested.

If, however, Kiara had been unhealthy (Question 15), medication may have been trialled while her nutritional status and safe swallowing was investigated.

Measurement of Drooling

The accurate measurement of drooling is difficult; it can vary from day to day and activity to activity. For the most part, rating scales are used to assess the severity of the drooling. Here is an example of one scale used to rate the drooling that has been adapted from the scales used by Camp-Bruno, Winsberg, Green-Parsons, and Abrams (1989), and Thomas-Stonell and Greenberg (1988).

The Saliva Loss Rating Scale

This scale has two parts: Frequency and Severity.

Frequency
1. No drooling—dry
2. Minimal drooling—small amount
3. Occasional drooling—on and off all day
4. Frequent drooling but not profuse
5. Frequent drooling and profuse
6. Constant drooling, always wet

Severity
1. Dry—never drools
2. Mild—only the lips are wet
3. Moderate—wet on the lips and the chin
4. Severe—drools to the extent the clothes are damp
5. Profuse—clothing, hands, tray, and objects become wet

5. Profuse—clothing, hands, tray, and objects become wet

To use the scale:

1. At least two people should complete the scale daily. The scales should be scored separately and not involve discussion between the two scorers.

2. If possible, the client should be encouraged or assisted to complete the scale daily (that is, a self-report). A second person who knows the client well and has daily contact should also complete the scale. It is advisable to complete the scale at the end of the day. Family members should be encouraged to complete the scale, especially on weekends and holidays. Rating can continue during the treatment and at periodic times after intervention (for example, every six months after surgery).

3. Complete scale daily for at least five to ten days.

4. Draw up a chart for easy recording. On this chart record the number that corresponds to the frequency and severity of drooling (see Rating Scale Chart, page 26). Please note that when using the rating scale reliability and validity measures need to be included.

An alternative rating scale is suggested by Thomas-Stonell and Greenberg (1988).

Severity

1. Dry: never drools
2. Mild: only the lips are wet
3. Moderate: wet on the lips and chin
4. Severe: drools to the extent that clothing becomes damp
5. Profuse: clothing, hands, tray, and objects become wet

Frequency

1. Never drools
2. Occasional drooling
3. Frequent drooling
4. Constant drooling
- The client is rated by a consensus judgment of prime caregivers and therapists.
- The drooling rankings from both scales are added together to make a combined drooling score.

Saliva Control Assessment

September 1990
Saliva Control Group
Melbourne, Australia.

Please answer the following questions. Write any comments where necessary.

Name _____

Date _____ Date of Birth _____

1. Drooling began after an accident or illness   _____

    Has always had a problem with dribbling   _____

    Drooling has improved   _____

    Drooling has worsened   _____

2. Can keep the head up?   Yes ____ No ____

    Limited Skills   _____

3. Frequently sits with head down?   Yes ____ No ____

4. Is mouth habitually open?   Yes ____ No ____

5. Person can hold lips together indefinitely   _____

    with ease for a limited time   _____

    with effort for a limited time   _____

    can bring lips together very briefly _____

    is unable to bring lips together   _____

6. Can suck through a short regular straw   _____

    with ease   _____

    with difficulty   _____

    not at all   _____

7. Can lick food off lips   _____

8. Can pucker lip   _____

Copyright © 1993 by Communication Skill Builders, a division of The Psychological Corporation / All rights reserved
1-800-228-0752 / ISBN 0761678956

Saliva Control Assessment (continued)

9. Chewing is up and down only _____

    Tends to suck food _____

10. Types of food able to eat _____

    pureed _____

    mashed _____

    chopped food with lumps _____

    whole foods (for example, carrots, steak, raw vegetables) _____

11. Shows awareness of saliva on lips _____

    on chin _____

12. Reacts strongly to acidity (e.g., fruit juice) _____

    Reacts strongly to temperature (e.g., hot/cold) _____

    Reacts strongly to certain food consistencies (e.g., lumps) _____

13. How often does the person swallow in 10 minutes? _____

14. Closes lips during swallowing _____

    Tongue protrudes during swallowing _____

    Uses gravity (puts head back) to swallow _____

    Can swallow saliva on demand _____

    Understands the concept "swallow" _____

15. Is usually healthy _____

16. Has frequent blocked or runny nose   _____

        Has asthma   _____

        Has allergies (specify)   _____

17. Is regular medication necessary?   _____

        If so, what is it?   _____

        Have you noticed if the
medication has any effect
on drooling?   _____

_____

_____

18. Are there any behaviors that might increase
the drooling—for example, spitting, hands
in the mouth, sucks objects continually?
Please comment.   _____

_____

_____

19. Please include a dental report of occlusion
and oral hygiene. If none is available,
please describe the state of the teeth
and gums.

Observation of Saliva Control Checklist

Please answer yes/no or add comments to all of the following.

a. Drooling is present all of the time. _____

b. Drooling is most obvious when tired/unwell or has a cold. _____

c. Drooling seems to change with the weather. _____

d. Drooling varies from day to day. _____

e. Drooling is more noticeable at a particular time of day or month (e.g., afternoon at menstruation). _____

f. Drooling is mostly present after eating or drinking. _____

g. Drooling is mostly present when concentrating on an activity (e.g., watching TV). _____

h. Shows awareness of the drooling. _____

i. Swallows frequently (e.g., once a minute). _____

j. Can stay dry but needs constant reminders. _____

k. Can keep chin dry by wiping without being prompted. _____

l. Wipes chin only when asked. _____

m. Attempts to wipe chin but needs assistance. _____

n. Saliva pours out of the mouth at intervals. _____

o. Saliva is continuously present on lips and chin. _____

p. Saliva is mostly apparent on the lips with an occasional wet chin. _____

q. The saliva has an unpleasant odor. _____

r. Describe the saliva flow, e.g., continuous wet stream, only on one side, falls on schoolwork, and so on. _____

s. Needs to change clothes/bibs _____ times a day.

Rating Scale Chart

Name of Client _____

Date	Frequency	Severity	Initials of Rater

Saliva Control Assessment—Post Surgery

Period of time since operation: 1 month   6 months
                                  12 months   2 years
                                  Other (state period)

Client's name _____ D.O.B. _____

Date of surgery _____

Name of surgeon _____

Place of surgery _____

Length of hospitalization _____

Type of surgery _____

Any complications? _____

Have any previous saliva control
    operations been performed?   ☐ Yes   ☐ No

If yes: operation performed _____ Date _____

OBJECTIVE MEASUREMENT: Date of observation: _____

Ratings of drooling severity

	FREQUENCY	SEVERITY
Pre-operative measurements:	1 _____	1 _____
	2 _____	2 _____
	3 _____	3 _____
	4 _____	4 _____
	5 _____	5 _____
Post-operative measurements:	1 _____	1 _____
	2 _____	2 _____
	3 _____	3 _____
	4 _____	4 _____
	5 _____	5 _____

Saliva Control Assessment—Post Surgery *(continued)*

DESCRIPTIVE MEASUREMENT: Date of observation: _____

Perceived severity of saliva problem:

☐ MILD   ☐ MODERATE   ☐ SEVERE

☐ Present in period of concentration only

☐ Consistently present

☐ Can control in times of social necessity

Comment on perceived change in severity since operation _____

_____

_____

_____

_____

Quality of saliva

☐ Clear   ☐ Opaque
☐ Yellowish   ☐ Very watery
☐ Slightly sticky   ☐ Thick and mucousy
☐ No odor   ☐ Sometimes offensive
☐ Offensive odor   ☐ Frothy
☐ Moist chin   ☐ Falls in drops
☐ Falls in strings   ☐ Requires firm wipe
☐ Requires repeated and persistent wiping

Comment on perceived change in quality of saliva since operation:

_____

_____

_____

_____

Dentition

Bite: ☐ Normal ☐ Class 1 ☐ Class 2 ☐ Class 3

Gums: ☐ Healthy ☐ Diseased

Oral hygiene: ☐ Good ☐ Adequate ☐ Poor

Caries: _____

_____

Comment on any change in state of dentition since operation: _____

_____

_____

_____

General

Have there been any ear infections or ear problems since the operation?

_____

_____

_____

Please describe: _____

_____

Has there been any change in the desire for food or fluids since the operation? Please describe: _____

_____

_____

Oral Secretion Assessment Form

Date: _____

Name: _____

Key

N = normal
D = dry mouth
R = ropy/thick saliva
W = watery saliva

Qualifications

\+ excessive
\++ very excessive

Pre/Post Trial

Date:	Breakfast		Mid-morning		Lunch		Mid-afternoon		Dinner		Evening	
	Before	After	Before	After	Before	After	Before	After	Before	After	Before	After

Instructions

1. Fill in the form on three days in one week (the days need not be successive).

2. Evaluate oral secretions before and after eating and/or drinking (if you don't eat or drink anything at any of the assessment times, simply indicate that before space).

3. Use the abbreviations listed above when appropriate; quantify your evaluation with plus signs. In some cases two separate symbols may be needed (for example, "D" and "R").

4. Don't take any medication aimed at altering secretions during the pre-trial evaluation week.

Chapter 3 — APPROACHES TO THE MANAGEMENT OF DROOLING

After the evaluation, an appropriate program is implemented from the treatment options listed below:

Eating and Drinking Skills
Oral-Facial Facilitation
Behavior Management
Appliances
Medications Used in the Control of Oro-Pharyngeal Secretions
The Surgical Management of Drooling

Eating and Drinking Skills (Hilary Johnson)

Frequently drooling occurs where eating and drinking skills are either not fully established or where skills have been lost—for example, after a stroke (CVA). There are many articles and books written on the subject; for further information see the reference list, page 83. The further development of eating and drinking skills might be indicated by answers to Questions 6-10 in the Saliva Control Assessment.

To maximize eating and drinking skills:

1. Obtain a full assessment of eating and drinking skills.

2. Follow a program to assist in maximizing those skills.

3. Where there is a remaining drooling problem, ascertain whether certain substances/foods are contributing to it. For instance, acidic fruit drinks or alcohol can stimulate the saliva while other substances can cause a person to have a dry mouth. Help the person who drools to establish any external factors that may contribute to the drooling in order for the person to most effectively control saliva.

Oral-Facial Facilitation *(Amanda Scott/Gloria Staios)* _____

Various techniques of oral-facial facilitation have been developed with the aim of improving oral function and therefore increasing the ability to control saliva. Drooling often occurs as a result of poor oral-motor control, a decrease in the frequency of spontaneous swallowing, and/or a reduction in the sensory awareness necessary for swallowing. Answers to Questions 4, 5, 11, 12, 13, and 14 on the Saliva Control Assessment may indicate the need for oral-facial facilitation. Techniques used to improve these conditions include the use of icing, brushing, vibration, and manipulation through tapping, stroking, and patting. These techniques attempt to normalize muscle tone and to provide intensive sensory input aimed at increasing oral awareness and discrimination. Examples of programs using these techniques are outlined further in this chapter.

Oral-facial facilitation techniques have been used to improve control of saliva with people who have hypertonic (high tone) and hypotonic (low tone, flaccid) muscles. This occurs in the following clinical population groups:

- children with cerebral palsy and other neurological conditions.
- children with intellectual impairment.
- children with low muscle tone, usually associated with developmental delay.
- adults with cerebral palsy and other developmental neurological conditions.
- adults with acquired neurological impairment such as cerebral vascular accident, and adults with a progressive neurological impairment, amyotrophic lateral sclerosis, or multiple sclerosis.

Clinical experience has shown that oral-facial facilitation techniques vary in their effectiveness. It is therefore appropriate to trial these techniques before introducing them into the daily routine. It is also important to introduce these techniques gradually in order to build up tolerance to the sensory input, because some individuals may initially find the stimulation aversive.

Physical Positioning

Before using any of these techniques, the individual receiving treatment should be positioned appropriately. When sitting it is important to ensure that the shoulder girdle, trunk, and pelvis are stable, and that the feet are flat on the floor or footplates of the wheelchair. The back of the neck should be straight, with the chin slightly tucked (see figures 4 and 5).

With severely disabled individuals who are confined to bed, it is important that they are in a comfortable and well-supported position, sitting up as much as possible.

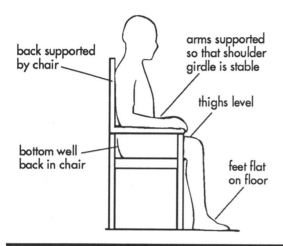

back supported by chair

arms supported so that shoulder girdle is stable

thighs level

bottom well back in chair

feet flat on floor

Figure 4. Correct positioning for oral facial facilitation: stable shoulder girdle, pelvis and trunk.

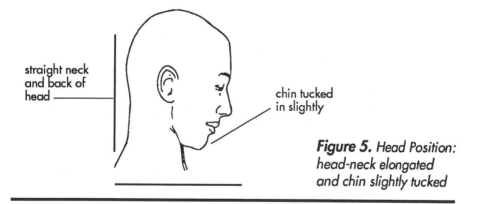

straight neck and back of head

chin tucked in slightly

Figure 5. Head Position: head-neck elongated and chin slightly tucked

Once the individual is in a stable and comfortable position, one (or a combination) of the following programs can be tried.
1. Icing
2. Brushing
3. Vibration
4. Manipulation
5. Oral-motor/sensory exercises

Icing (see figure 6).

The application of ice directly over the target muscle has been found to normalize muscle tone in some individuals, thereby improving oral-motor function and enhancing sensory awareness. To maximize the effectiveness of this procedure, an oral activity such as eating or exercises should directly follow icing. The effects of icing are immediate and may last between 5 and 30 minutes.

Application of ice to the face:

- apply firm even pressure along the muscle in the direction of the muscle movement.
- ice facial areas first, proceed to mouth, and then inside mouth.
- to normalize tone in the tongue, mouth, and pharynx, an ice cube can be sucked. Ensure that there are no sharp edges (Langley 1987).
- ice should be applied for three to ten seconds, depending on the tolerance level of the individual and the effectiveness of the procedure.
- ice along the cheeks (buccinator muscle).
- ice over the masseter muscle.
- ice around the lips (orbicularis oris muscle).

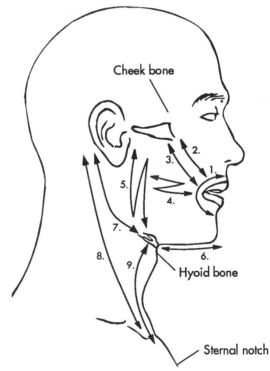

Figure 6. Diagram for sequence and direction of icing and brushing techniques

It has been found that ice helps to stimulate delayed or absent swallow reflex. (Logeman 1983)

Application of ice to stimulate swallow reflex.

The following are strategies that have been found to be useful.

- apply an ice pack to the neck at the level of the thyroid cartilage.
- apply ice directly to the thyroid notch.
- apply ice to the anterior faucial arches (see figure 7) and immediately above the uvula using a frozen wetted cotton swab or chilled laryngeal mirror (to be used only if tone is normal or low).

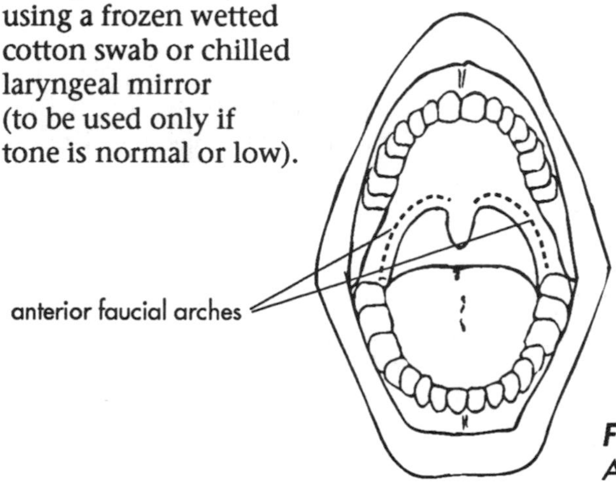

anterior faucial arches

Figure 7.
Anterior faucial arches

When using these icing procedures, the following considerations should be taken into account:

- ice facial areas first, proceed to mouth and then inside mouth.
- ice can be a noxious stimulus that may lead to seizures in some individuals with epilepsy, or increase spasticity and rigidity in others.
- ice may not be effective and may cause great discomfort for individuals who are hypersensitive or who are sensory defensive.
- ice may cause "ice burns," evident by reddening of the skin; therefore, care must be taken during application.
- sucking ice is not recommended for individuals with severe tongue thrust because it reinforces the thrusting pattern (Gallender 1979).
- icing in the region of the carotid sinus (behind the left ear) should be avoided in individuals with severe cardiac problems.

The following ideas for handling the ice have been found useful:

- small ice cubes (made from water, as sweet/citrus fruit juice cubes increase salivation).
- iced wetted cotton swabs (placed in individual fingers of a surgical glove and frozen).
- crushed ice in a disposable surgical glove (fingers can be used like a frozen treat).
- frozen fruit juice on a stick (molds are available in supermarkets).
- ice sticks (water frozen in a plastic straw). Push 2 cm of the ice out of the straw and apply to the desired area holding the straw firmly (Morris and Klein 1987).
- a small long-handled laryngeal mirror that has been placed in ice water is especially useful for cold stimulation to faucial arches (Logeman 1983). Always be wary of putting objects in the mouth if the person has a strong reflexive bite.

Brushing

Brushing is another procedure reported to normalize tone and increase sensory awareness. The effects of brushing are said to occur 20 to 30 minutes after the procedure (Langley 1987). Brushing should take place a half hour before a meal, or a half hour before an oral activity/exercise.

Methods for brushing include:

Manual brushing: For manual brushing use a medium-sized camel hair paintbrush. Use light rapid stroking along the muscle in the direction of the muscle movement. It is recommended that brushing not take place for more than three seconds per muscle (Langley 1987).

Fast rotary brushing/battery-operated brushing: Provide firm, even brushing to the muscle in the direction of the muscle movement. This method is considered to be more effective than manual brushing for stimulating hypotonic (flaccid) muscles.

Procedure for brushing (refer to figure 6, page 34, for sequence and direction of brushing technique):

- brush along the cheeks (buccinator)
- brush biting and inside surface of teeth
- brush tongue, lips, and cheeks to stimulate muscle tone
- brush lateral borders of tongue for improved chewing

- an electric toothbrush can be introduced with the above regime, and may be particularly useful for asymmetrical oral-facial structures, if the individual can tolerate it

When using these brushing procedures the following considerations should be taken into account:

- introduce brushing to the face first, proceed to the mouth, and then inside mouth.
- do not stimulate the temporalis muscle as this will result in jaw retraction (Gallender 1979).
- monitor the reaction to brushing and grade the stimulation accordingly.

Vibration

Vibration aims to increase proprioceptive input and facilitate more normal tone. Clinically it has been found to be more effective than brushing, perhaps due to its more intense stimulation. Although considered to be effective for stimulating hypotonic muscles, it has also been found useful for those with hypertonic muscles.

If the individual reacts strongly to vibration applied to the oral area, develop tolerance by first applying the stimulus to other parts of the body (for example, arms, backs of hands) for brief intervals (Grant 1982).

Procedure for application of vibration (manual and battery operated):

- apply vibration directly to the target muscles in the direction of the movement for approximately 6 to 10 seconds (refer to figure 6, page 34).
- vibrate along the cheeks (buccinator muscles)
- vibrate over masseter muscles
- vibrate around mouth (orbicularis oris muscles)
- vibrate under the chin
- apply vibration directly above the thyroid notch and over thyroid lamina to stimulate a swallow reflex and cough
- vibrate the area from either side of the nostrils area in a downward direction to the bottom of the upper lip (figure 8) to decrease upper lip retraction (Morris and Klein 1987).

Using index finger and middle finger parted, simultaneously vibrate from sides of nostrils to upper lip

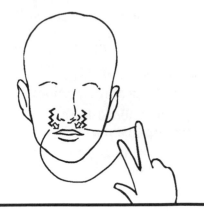

Figure 8: *Vibration between nose and upper lip*

- using the index finger, vibrate on the center of the tongue in a downward direction to flatten it. Stroke the tongue in forward direction as index finger is withdrawn to decrease tongue retraction
- vibrate the cheek (figure 9) and gently move forward while grasping the cheek between the index finger (inside the mouth) and middle finger (along the cheek) to decrease hypertonicity and reduce upper lip retraction (Morris and Klein 1987).

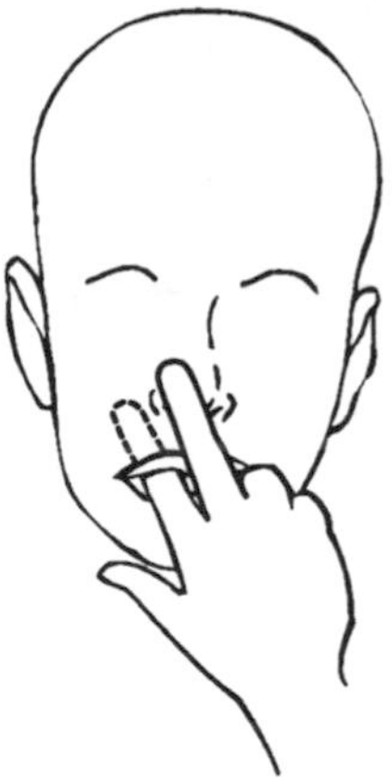

Figure 9. *Vibration of the cheek using index and middle fingers*

When using vibration the following considerations should be taken into account:

- ensure that vibration is not too intense, as this may result in an undesired increase in tone, rigidity, or extensor spasm (discontinue if vibration results in an increase in hypertonicity)
- use with caution if individual has epilepsy
- individuals with hydrocephalus should not receive this treatment
- vibration inside the mouth is not appropriate if the individual has a tonic bite reflex

Manipulation

Manipulation techniques such as tapping, stroking, and patting are applied directly to the muscles, using fingertips only. Firm even pressure should be applied throughout the procedures. A quick stretch along the muscle fibers may be useful for stimulating hypotonic muscles. Manipulation procedures are useful not only for their direct effect on facilitating normal movement patterns but also for improving oral function through increased oral awareness and discrimination.

Manipulation procedures:

- stroke face firmly in a downward direction
- wipe face with a towel, maintaining constant even pressure. This is particularly useful for individuals who are hypersensitive and have lip retraction due to increased tone (Morris and Klein 1987).
- flick the cheeks firmly but gently in an upward direction
- pull bottom lip up flush against upper lip
- pull tongue (in a piece of gauze) and shake it gently before returning to mouth. If necessary, facilitate lip closure afterwards.
- tap under the chin in an upward direction to facilitate an increase in tone in hypotonic tongue and to improve tongue stability
- tap tongue, cheeks, and around mouth in a regular, rhythmical manner. This is particularly useful for a hypotonic face. Tap directly around the tempero-mandibular joint for increased jaw stability.
- stroke the upper and lower gums, using firm even pressure. Grade the pressure as necessary if the individual is hypersensitive.
- stroke the tongue in a forward direction and the inside of the cheeks in a downward direction, using firm even pressure, to decrease tone in hypertonic muscles
- make small circular movements around the mouth and under the chin. Do not press the larynx.
- lift larynx from below the thyroid cartilage to stimulate a reflex swallow. This procedure is useful to facilitate a swallow in those who do not have a spontaneous swallow.

Discontinue these techniques if stimulation results in hypertonicity in the oral-facial area or other parts of the body.

Oral-Motor Sensory Exercises

The following are suggested exercises and activities that may be incorporated into an individual's program to improve oral-motor function, with the ultimate aim of improving saliva control. These exercises should immediately follow oral-facial facilitation techniques.

Lip Exercises

- make faces in mirror making various shapes with lips (for example, smiling, pursing, etc.)
- hold spatula or piece of paper between lips
- use a wide-diameter straw to suck up thickened fluids (for example, pureed apple or tissue paper) and blow items such as paper and cotton wool (facilitation of lip closure may be necessary). These exercises also require adequate velo-pharyngeal (soft palate against the pharyngeal wall) closure.
- place foods such as jam on the top lip and encourage removal with the bottom lip

Tongue Exercises

- Encourage food to be licked from specific sites using the tongue only. Place the food (for example, jam/honey) at various sites inside the mouth and on and around the lips.
- Encourage the person to lick food from a plate or off the end of a spatula held in front of the mouth. (An ice-cream stick can be very motivating!)
- Encourage the person to lick envelopes, stickers, lollipops, and so on. (Facilitation of tongue movements may be necessary for some of these exercises. This can be done by moving the tongue with a craft stick or your finger.)

Sensory Exercises

- apply different textures to the face, such as shaving cream, fur, textured plastic/rubber items, rice, soap suds
- for children, encourage oral exploration and mouthing of toys of various textures. (Ensure that the toys are non-toxic and are not small enough to be inhaled.)

Devising an Oral-Facial Facilitation Program for Your Client

When designing an oral-facial facilitation program for your client it is important to consider the following:

1. a trial of facilitation techniques.
2. the frequency, length, and timing of the program.
3. the training of the client, caregiver(s), and significant others implementing the program.
4. monitoring the effectiveness of the program.

Do not try all five techniques at once. Choose one technique at a time and evaluate its effectiveness. A trial of three sessions should be adequate to determine this.

Carefully grade the stimulation to increase tolerance, as some individuals may be sensitive to intense stimulation. You may present stimulation to other parts of the body as a preliminary introduction to the quality and intensity of the stimulus prior to presentation to the oral-facial area.

If, after a reasonable trial, the results are minimal or not significant, discontinue the trial and introduce another of the techniques. Once the trials have been completed choose the technique that was most effective, or a combination of effective techniques to implement as a part of the individual's daily routine.

Implementation of the Program

Once the program has been devised and implementation begins, it must be carefully monitored and regularly reviewed. The program should be implemented at least three times daily, and initially should be introduced for short periods until there is an increase in tolerance to the stimulation.

Take advantage of daily routines such as mealtimes and teethbrushing times to implement some of the techniques which have been outlined. Not only does this allow for treatment to take place in natural situations, but it also facilitates the consistent implementation of the program at regular and routine intervals. Utilizing the concepts of "facials" and "putting on make-up" are useful ways of implementing a more relaxed approach to sensory stimulation.

Training

Caregivers and significant others should be trained in the implementation of the oro-facial facilitation program. They should also be trained to observe and record the effects of the program and provide appropriate reinforcement to the individual receiving treatment.

The following program is an example of how various oral-facial facilitation techniques can be used in combination. This program is adapted from a workshop presented by Margaret Rood in London, Ontario, Canada, in 1973.

The following equipment is required:
- battery brush or medium-sized paintbrush
- iced cotton balls or narrow ice molds
- small hand towel/face cloth
- 1 mm-wide stainless steel blade
- plastic straw about 3/4-mm wide

1. Pressure and stretching around the mouth (figure 10). Avoid touching the lips.

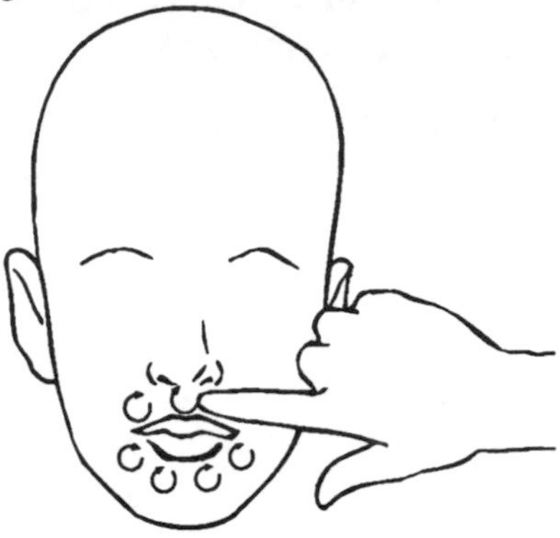

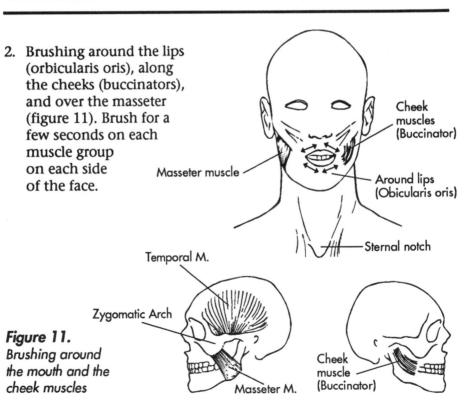

Figure 10. *Pressure and stretching around the mouth*

2. Brushing around the lips (orbicularis oris), along the cheeks (buccinators), and over the masseter (figure 11). Brush for a few seconds on each muscle group on each side of the face.

Cheek muscles (Buccinator)

Masseter muscle

Around lips (Obicularis oris)

Sternal notch

Temporal M.

Zygomatic Arch

Figure 11. *Brushing around the mouth and the cheek muscles*

Masseter M.

Cheek muscle (Buccinator)

3. Thirty seconds later apply ice with frozen treat. Mop dry after each swipe to stop the drips.

4. Repeat pressure and stretching around the mouth (orbicularis oris).

5. Walk stainless steel blade back along tongue (figure 12) to the beginning of the gag reflex, three times. (Avoid eliciting the gag reflex).

6. Slip the iced cotton swab from tip of tongue to the back along the central groove.

7. Swiftly stroke ice up across the sternal notch.

8. Using baby apple sauce or soft ice cream, have the client suck the food up a straw or from the tip of a spoon, several times.

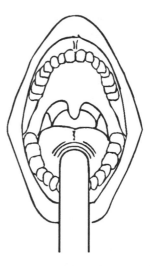

Figure 12. Walking stainless steel blade on the tongue

Conclusion

It has been shown that oral-facial facilitation techniques are effective in reducing but not eliminating drooling (Strawbridge, Domaracki, and Sisson 1990). These techniques serve to improve oral-motor function through intensive sensory stimulation. They also increase oral awareness and discrimination.

When developing an oral-facial facilitation program it is important to trial and evaluate the effectiveness of the techniques implemented and modify the program according to the responses and needs of the client.

Behavior Management (Bronwen Jones) _____

Learning about Saliva Control

Possible candidates for behavioral therapy may have been identified by answers to Questions 4, 5, 11, 12, 13, 14, and 18 on the Saliva Control Assessment form.

Behavioral therapy, or the learning of a new behavior, can be the first step in therapy for saliva control, or it can be utilized in conjunction with another therapy (medication, for example). Successful behavioral therapy requires commitment from all parties involved.

In deciding which clients will benefit most from a behavioral program for saliva control, the answer is not clear cut. By definition, a behavioral program implies the learning and integration of a new skill, and the literature on saliva control suggests that success with a behavioral program relies on certain basic cognitive ability. The actual research has shown varying degrees of success with a wide variety of individuals, methods, and intensities of treatment.

Behavioral therapy must be seen in the context of a continuum of learning theory (see figure 13). This has two sides.

The right-hand side of the continuum is the learning and integration of a new behavior because it has positive and perceivable consequences for the learner. This results in consistent use of the new behavior because the learner is internally motivated to use the new learning.

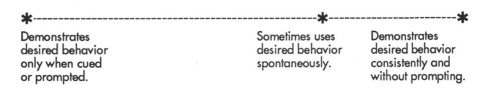

| Demonstrates desired behavior only when cued or prompted. | Sometimes uses desired behavior spontaneously. | Demonstrates desired behavior consistently and without prompting. |

Figure 13. Continuum of learning theory

The left side of the continuum is where learning theory has been applied, but individuals may not yet have perceived any reason for learning a new behavior. They may have learned the behavior or skill and used it in some situations or with some cuing, but they have not learned that the behavior has positive consequences for them and they do not choose to use their skill consistently.

Many people would argue that people whose behaviors mee[t] [cri]teria of the left side of the continuum have been unsuccessf[ul] behavioral program. Rather, this may be seen as success in t[he] compensatory behavior, but a further program may be require[d] [to] motivate the person to internalize the skills. For some people, the connection between a behavior and a desirable consequence cannot be internalized because they do not have a full understanding of cause and effect.

The indicators for success with a program lie in tailoring the treatment to suit the skills, motivation, interests, and cognitive level of each individual. Ensuring that goals are clear, and that people involved in the implementation understand their roles and are committed to the goals are also vital to success.

What is a behavioral learning program?

A behavioral learning program is designed to increase, decrease, or stop the occurrence of a specific behavior. *Example:* A program aimed at losing weight may include learning to decrease eating behaviors and/or to increase exercise behavior.

Similarly, a saliva control program may aim to increase swallowing behavior, decrease open-mouth behavior, or stop "hands-in-mouth" behavior. Behavioral learning programs consist of specific steps no matter what behavior is being targeted for new learning.

Which behavior do I want to change?

Specific behaviors that have been targeted in saliva control programs are:

- Learning to maintain better head posture (Thomas-Stonell and Greenberg 1988).
- Learning lip closure and jaw stability (Helfrich-Miller, Rector, and Straka 1986; Harris and Purdy 1987; Thomas-Stonell and Greenberg 1988).
- Learning more effective swallowing (including chewing, eating, and intra-oral pressure) (Thorbecke and Jackson 1982; Dunn, Cunningham, and Blackman 1987; Koheil, Sochaniwskyj, Bablich, Kenny, and Milner 1987).
- Learning effective chin wiping (Drabman, Cordua Y Cruz, Ross, and Lynd 1979; Rapp 1980).

There may be a variety of behaviors contributing to the problem, so it is important to describe the behaviors carefully and decide which one is contributing most to the problem. Example: Bernard is a young man with a severe intellectual disability. He has poor oral muscle tone which results in poor lip closure and inefficient swallowing. He also has a habit of putting his fisted right hand into his mouth as part of his self-stimulatory behavior. During observations of Bernard in several situations, his loss of saliva was mild when his hands were occupied and moderate to severe when he had his hand in his mouth. It was decided that a behavioral program to reduce his "hand-to-mouth" behavior was the most appropriate.

Measuring the Behavior

To determine whether the learning program has been effective, it is important to measure and describe so that you have a baseline against which to measure change.

You may choose to measure the behavior you wish to teach (for example, lips together) or the contingent behavior that is the presenting problem (that is, loss of saliva). If you choose to measure loss of saliva as the presenting problem, then you must be confident that the skill you choose to teach will help solve the problem. If you have taught the skill and there is no change in levels of saliva loss, then you may have chosen a behavior that was irrelevant to loss of saliva. You may need to teach more than one new skill to alleviate the problem (better head posture and more frequent swallowing), so measuring the saliva loss will give you the most information about which behavior is contributing most to the problem. (More information about measuring and describing techniques is provided in Chapter 2.)

Planning and Preparation

The planning stage may involve a team of people who know the person well (parents, teachers, friends, neighbors, siblings, co-workers, staff, work supervisors, etc.). This helps ensure that the most realistic assessment of the person's skills, motivation, interests, and cognitive level are taken into account in the planning.

Defining Goals

In planning goals, not only does the skill to be learned need to be identified, but also the situations in which the skill or behavior should or should not occur. The goals must be:

Objective: Describing observable characteristics of skill/behavior. For example, Terry will learn to close his lips together and swallow (with lips together) when requested.

Clear: Unambiguous

Complete: Delineate boundary conditions. Example: Carla will learn to lift her head to an upright and midline position when staff say, "Head up, Carla," only when Carla is seated in her postured work chair.

It is important that specific, observable skills/behaviors become the target of the learning program rather than the global idea of "drooling." A specified behavior is much easier to deal with than general impressions.

Deciding on a key worker

Behavioral programs require consistency and persistence. There must be at least one person who can spend time with the client on a daily basis and is prepared to be persistent in the administration of the program. This person needs to be integrally involved in the planning and setting of goals so that there is a personal investment in the outcomes. The key person may require training and access to other members of the planning team for advice, problem solving, and ongoing support.

This key person may be a teacher, teacher's aide, parent, co-worker, supervisor, or any person who understands the program goals and is able to spend time administering the program. The key person may need training in:

- observing behaviors and responses in order to provide appropriate feedback.
- differentiating responses so that the "best" skill/behavior can be shaped and rewarded.
- rewarding and responding at the appropriate time and with the "right amount" of reward.
- measuring and describing. The key worker must not rely totally on human judgment or unstructured impressions. Actual frequency of behaviors is often misjudged depending on the mood or the memory of the person reporting if complete, objective records are not maintained.

Evaluation

In planning the program, it is important to have ongoing evaluation built in as part of the procedure. This usually involves measuring changes in the frequency of target skills, or changes in the contingent behaviors. The information obtained in these measurements may indicate that goals need to be altered. For example, if teaching the reduction of "hands-in-mouth" behavior as a new skill was having no impact on the level of saliva loss, then either the relevance of the skill or the effectiveness of the teaching would need to be revised.

Motivation to Learn, or "Different Strokes for Different Folks"

Appropriate and motivating consequences or reinforcers can make or break a program. This is one reason why it is important to know the person well in order to assess what in particular will be a motivating reinforcer.

Example: Filipo loves physical contact and interacting with people. Verbal praise and a pat on the back are appropriate reinforcers for Filipo.

Julia doesn't like being touched and doesn't enjoy being with people. Filipo's reinforcers would not be rewarding for Julia.

Types of consequences/reinforcers: There are two main types of reinforcement: positive and negative.

A *positive reinforcer* is an event presented after a behavior has been performed that increases the frequency of that particular behavior.

Examples:

- Julio lifts up his head and his mother responds by turning on the television. Julio lifts his head more often.

- Sally closes her lips and swallows and her workshop supervisor responds by smiling at her and saying how pretty Sally looks today. Sally's lip closure increases and she swallows more often.

A *negative reinforcer* is an event that is removed after a behavior has been performed that increases the frequency of that behavior.

For the purposes of saliva control programs, positive reinforcers are easier to plan for and administer than negative reinforcers, but occasionally a negative reinforcer may be appropriate.

Examples:

- Spiros wears a lip sensor that emits an unpleasant squeal if his lips are parted. When he closes his lips, the noise stops. Spiros doesn't like the noise, so he keeps his lips together.

- Bronwen is embarrassed by her mother's constant comments on her saliva and her patronizing wiping of Bronwen's chin. Bronwen begins swallowing more when she is with her mother and generally stays dry. Mother's comments and wipings cease.

Which reinforcer is most powerfully motivating?

Reinforcers can be further categorized into primary, secondary (or conditioned), and generalized conditioned reinforcers.

Primary reinforcers involve basic physical needs and sensations: for example, food, drink (positive reinforcers), or shock, loud noise (negative reinforcers).

Secondary reinforcers have to be conditioned (for example, praise, money, and so on.)

Generalized conditioned reinforcers have a variety of reinforcing events contributing to their value and are generally the most useful, if they are motivating to the client (for example, attention).

Examples:
- tokens, chips (money can buy a variety of rewarding events such as TV, snacks, outings)
- attention or approval may bring associated physical contact, praise, smiles, and so on

The best reinforcement is the motivation that comes from achieving the skill and all the positive responses that occur with new learning (for example, praise, independence).

Reinforcers can also consist of food/consumables, social high-probability behaviors, feedback, and tokens. Table 1 lists examples of each of these reinforcers and lists pros and cons of the different types of reinforcers.

Schedules—It's all in the timing

Once the goals have been set and the reinforcement type decided upon, a schedule of reinforcement must be planned. There are many ways of administering the reinforcements, and the schedule may need to change during different parts of the program.

Continuous reinforcement consists of a simple schedule in which reinforcement is given each time the desired behavior occurs. While a behavior is developing, continuous reinforcement helps the person to perform the behavior at a higher rate. (Behaviors that have been continuously reinforced also deteriorate quickly when the reinforcement is removed.)

Intermittent reinforcement is when the reinforcement is delivered only after the desired behavior has occurred several times. On an intermittent schedule, occurrence of the behavior continues for a longer period of time even after the reinforcement has ceased.

Table 1: List of Reinforcers

TYPE OF REINFORCER	SAMPLES/IDEAS	FOR	AGAINST
Food consumables	lollipops, cookies, gum, drinks	• Paired with social so that the secondary reinforcer is built to a strong level.	• Dependent on deprivation state • Interrupts ongoing behavior • Difficult to give immediately • Ethical issues of depriving of food, etc. • May increase drooling
Social	verbal praise, attention physical contact (touching, pats, hand-holding), facial expression (smile, eye contact, nods, wink)	• Easily given • Portable • Naturally occurring • Generalized reinforcer	• May not be naturally reinforcing
High probability	Playing with friends, watching TV, listening to music, playing a game		• Ethical issues of depriving a person who may already have limited control over life • Need a good cognitive understanding
Feedback	Can be paired with food, social, and so on, or can be given by itself • auditory (verbal, sound) • visual (scales, charts)	• Can be paired with a variety of other reinforcers • Can be naturally occurring and therefore maintain behavior	
Tokens	money, chips, stamps, buttons	• Very potent • Generalized reinforcer • Can be traded for a variety of motivating activities • Can be used to set up a delay in delivery of reward	• Hard to fade • Not naturally occurring • Not immediately rewarding—need to have ability to abstract to future event. Delay may not be understood.

Ratio schedule and *interval schedule* are both examples of intermittent reinforcement.

A ratio schedule consists of giving reinforcement only after the desired behavior has occurred a specified number of times. For example, Jitka receives one star on her chart for every five times she closes her lips and swallows.

An interval schedule is dependent upon the amount of time that passes before the reinforcement is given. Dina, for example, is given a token every 10 minutes if she sits up straight when her work supervisor looks over to check.

Interval schedules are easier to administer, but the individual's performance is usually higher under ratio schedules. Interval and ratio schedules may be fixed or variable. Variable ratio schedules are not easily extinguished and occur in real-life situations such as using slot machines or going fishing. Because there is no way of knowing when the reward is going to happen, the behavior continues at a high level (continuing to put money in the slot machine, waiting for a win, or continuing to throw the fishing line in, waiting for a bite).

Intermittent reinforcement has the benefits of:

- efficient use of reinforcers
- less time-consuming than administered continuous
- little risk of boredom or satiation with reinforcer

Generally, the best way to schedule reinforcement for a saliva control program is to start with a continuous (1:1) schedule until the desired behavior has been well established, then change to a ratio or interval schedule, and make the reinforcement more and more intermittent.

Shaping/Prompting/Fading

Not all people are going to be highly motivated to learn new behavior. Many people may learn the behavior during the program, but if they do not understand the benefits that the behavior provides, the behavior may not continue.

In providing a program, it is important to define how much assistance the client will be given to learn the behavior. This assistance may take the form of shaping a desired behavior, prompting the behavior to occur, and then fading out the prompts.

If motivation to learn the behavior and use the behavior is not evident at any stage, then fading out the prompts may not be a viable phase of the program.

Shaping is the reinforcement of a behavior that approximates the behavior to be learned. For example, if someone is learning to swallow more regularly, then reinforcing "lips together" in preparation for swallowing is a shaping procedure. Even if the person does not follow the lip closure with a swallow, an attempt is being made and must be reinforced as a precursor to the desired behavior. Reinforcement of approximations gradually ceases and the person is fully reinforced only for swallowing.

Prompting involves various ways of reminding the person to use the new skill/behavior. Prompts range from fully assisting the person physically to perform the skill through to a conditioned reminder that is unrelated to the skill (for example, swallowing on hearing a beep).

It is important to plan the sequence of prompts carefully so that the person can gradually become more independent in the learned skill use and not be reliant on continuous one-on-one prompting. For instance, if a person is learning a new head posture in order to control saliva, it is important that the prompts be reduced from, perhaps, full physical manipulation to attain correct head posture to a partial physical prompt, a gentle hand tap on the neck, for instance, then to a verbal/visual prompt of "head up." In reducing the strength of prompts, it is vital to ensure that success has been achieved at one level before moving on to a lesser prompt.

In planning a program, a fine line exists between giving too many prompts, so that the person becomes reliant on prompting to initiate the skill, and not enough prompts, so that the behavior is used too infrequently to become integrated as a new skill.

Fading is the process in which prompts gradually become fewer as the person internalizes use of the new behavior. With successful learning, fading of prompts should eventually become complete.

Fading needs to be gradual and prompts should be minimal, or have ceased by the end of training.

Generalization and Maintenance

Generalization of a skill may become necessary in a behavioral learning program for saliva control.

If a skill has been learned and practiced in one setting, it may or may not be used automatically in a different setting. For instance, someone may learn to stay dry in a social setting (for example, out shopping with friends), but may not transfer this skill to daily activities at a day-care center. A specific part of the program (or of a transfer program) may be designed to help generalize the use of a new skill in a variety of settings. Generalization may need to occur across places, times, or with various people.

Maintenance: So, you've administered a teaching program; your client has learned a new skill; you've faded your prompts; and the client is dry. Two weeks later, you see your client with a wet chin. What went wrong? Maybe the new skill had not really been internalized, or maybe the reinforcers weren't occurring regularly enough in the natural environment.

Follow-up and maintenance programs need to be planned for if you expect long-term success. Everyone needs support and encouragement. Maintenance may mean as little as regular meetings and pep talks to reinforce new learning.

Maintenance can occur in a self-help group to discuss problem times and to encourage people to maintain skill levels. Follow-up programs may be offered periodically to remind people of their skills. Maintenance of skills will be vastly different from person to person, so opportunities to revise and maintain must remain flexible. It may be wise to assign one person to monitor maintenance of the skills and report back on whether further intervention is required.

Examples of Behavioral Programs

Behavior Program 1: Learning a New Head Posture.

Client:
Doug is a 35-year-old man with cerebral palsy who works in a sheltered employment setting.

Persons Responsible:
Direct supervisor and speech-language pathologist.

Behavior to be learned:
To keep his head upright and in the midline in order to reduce saliva loss.

Goal:
For Doug to keep his head upright and in midline when he is seated at his workbench, which is angled so that his work is at eye level.

Measurement/Evaluation Schedule:

- Week 1. Direct supervisor gives Doug new work or removes work he has completed approximately every ten minutes. Direct supervisor to check head posture and praise correct posture or remind Doug and physically assist posture if it is not correct. Drooling is measured once a week.
- Week 2. Direct supervisor picks work up every 20 minutes and program continues.
- Week 3. Every 30 minutes. Charts progress.

Reinforcement:

- May need to physically assist lifting up chin.
- Prompt—Touch Doug on head to prompt head-up.
- Cue—When Doug looks at direct supervisor, supervisor lifts up own head.
- Praise, smiles.
- Monetary bonus at end of week for needing less than 20 percent reminders to maintain head posture.

Generalization:

Speech-language pathologist monitors Doug's head posture at lunch time in canteen in Week 4 of program. Week 6: Monitor head posture at a football game.

Maintenance:

Have a random week of charting and monitoring. Doug continues to receive wage bonus if he maintains head posture.

Behavior Program 2: Learning to Swallow More Frequently.

Client:

Jose is a 4-year-old boy with low oral tone who swallows infrequently.

Persons Responsible:

Jose's mother and speech-language pathologist.

Behavior to be learned:

To swallow more frequently in order to reduce saliva loss.

Goal:

For Jose to swallow once a minute when he is sitting quietly watching television.

Measurement/Evaluation Schedule:

Jose's saliva control to be rated five times over two weeks before the program begins. Jose's saliva control to be measured twice a week during the duration of the program and twice a week for one month after the program has ended. The program will last for one hour per day over three weeks. Total measurement/evaluation time—nine weeks.

Shape/Prompt/Cue/Fade:

Shape: Before the program begins, Jose will spend three 20-minute sessions with the speech-language pathologist learning how to swallow on request every 60 seconds. This can be done in a simple dice game where Jose has to swallow when he hears the buzzer or SLP's voice. Failure to swallow means Jose forfeits a turn. When Jose can swallow on request twenty times in twenty minutes, the program can begin.

Prompt: When Jose sits down to watch TV, his mother puts on a one-hour video cassette that has the SLP's voice instructing Jose to swallow and a beep accompanying the voice every 60 seconds.

Jose's mother will monitor his swallowing in Week 1, hours one, three, and five to shape his swallowing. In Week 2, she will monitor a random 30 minutes of hours six, eight, and ten.

In Week 3, Jose's mother will monitor a random 20 minutes of hours 12, 14, and 15.

Fade: When Jose is swallowing consistently 90 percent of the time in response to the tape, Jose will practice swallowing to a beep without the verbal reminder. During Week 3, the tape will be played for only thirty minutes of the hour that Jose is watching television.

Reinforcement:

Jose will receive a new toy car at the end of every week if he has achieved 90 percent swallowing during the time he was being monitored.

Mother will give Jose lots of praise for his swallowing and will make a chart to show him how many swallows he does each day, using colored stickers.

Generalization:

Jose can wear an ear plug attached to a beeper set to beep every 60 seconds. Jose may wear this for 30 minutes a day during different situations. After he has completed his program, the beep will act as a conditioned cue for him to swallow.

Maintenance:

Jose's mother will secretly observe his swallowing once a week for 15 minutes in a variety of situations. If Jose is swallowing less than once every 90 seconds, she may introduce the beeper each day for a week while he is watching television.

Appliances *(Libby Ferguson/Denise West)* _____

Abnormal muscle tone and movement of the tongue, lips, and cheeks often results in structural changes and difficulty attaining functional oral movements, such as lip closure, voluntary tongue movement, chewing, and swallowing. Various orthodontic appliances have been developed in an attempt to modify and improve oral motor function. These appliances vary in methods of attachment within the oral cavity and in the length of time they remain in the mouth.

All of these devices (except the Exeter lip sensor) need a dentist or suitably qualified personnel to ensure the appliances fit correctly. Regular checks of the mouth and appliance also mean that the family, caregiver, and person using the appliance will need to visit the dentist regularly.

Saliva control has rarely been the primary aim of clinical trials of orthodontic appliances. However, a reduction in drooling frequently has been reported in the literature. Most of the studies reported have been conducted by orthodontists and little attempt has been made to objectively measure drooling behavior. The relationship between saliva control and the fitting of orthodontic appliances has been researched infrequently.

When an orthodontic appliance for the purpose of saliva control is contemplated, the following considerations need to be addressed:

1. The person's ability to retain the appliance securely may vary due to:
   - dentition
   - oral muscle tone
   - intra-oral sensation
   - cooperation
   - comfort

2. The person's motivation and ability to comply with the program.

3. The availability of regular support and review by appropriate dental/orthodontic staff.

4. The person's physiological and behavioral ability to tolerate the appliance.

5. Age of the person.

Some of the advantages and disadvantages of the fitting of appliances for saliva control are presented in Table 2.

Table 2: Advantages and disadvantages of using oral appliances for saliva control

ADVANTAGES	DISADVANTAGES
• non-invasive (that is, does not involve drugs, surgery, or anesthesia).	• difficult retaining appliance in the mouth.
• some appliances are relatively inexpensive in terms of professional time, intervention, and purchase.	• some are expensive to trial in both materials and staff time.
	• may need a number of visits to the dentist/orthodontist.
• not costly.	• varying degrees of discomfort.
	• possibility of ulceration of oral structures.
• can result in improved oral-motor functioning and desirable structural modification.	• results of use of appliances are inadequately researched.
• usually temporary.	• some appliances may increase drooling initially.

The remainder of this section describes oral appliances that have been developed and can be used to improve oral motor function.

Myofunctional Appliance (figure 14)

This appliance is also referred to as the "chewing brush" or "ortho-munchie." It is an oral device consisting of a soft plastic mouth guard that fits over the upper and lower teeth. It has small protrusions to stimulate/massage the teeth and gums when chewed. The myofunctional appliance is actively chewed on for 20 to 40 minutes a day. It is designed to prevent tongue thrusting during use.

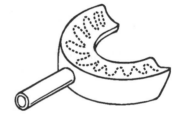

Figure 14.
Myofunctional appliance

The appliance is commercially available, comes in two sizes (small and large), and may be ordered with or without handles.

Claims have been made that the myofunctional appliance can:
- improve competence of facial muscles
- improve an open bite

- improve oral hygiene (removes plaque and promotes healthier oral tissues)
- correct developing malocclusions
- reduce tongue thrusting
- reduce drooling

The above claims have not yet been supported by published research articles in refereed journals.

The Palatal Training Appliance (p.t.a.) (figure 15)

This appliance was developed in England and was designed for people with hypernasal speech. It was found to improve swallowing performance and to decrease drooling.

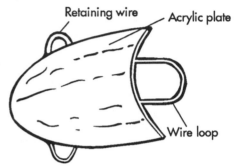

Figure 15. Palatal training appliance

The device is made from a loop of stainless steel wire that is bent into a "U" shape and made to conform to the vault of the resting soft palate. It does not touch the soft palate but touches the mucous membrane near the base of the uvula. It is worn on an acrylic plate or fitted to a denture. The wire loop is adjustable and needs to be securely fitted to prevent it from being swallowed by clients who have reduced palatal sensitivity.

The device is worn during the day but removed during sleep. An initial increase in salivation was reported. This was followed within a month by an increased rate of swallowing.

It has been suggested that the p.t.a. works by increasing tactile awareness or by adding an extra stimulus to trigger involuntary swallowing (increasing the stimulus to the afferent side of the reflex arc to the swallowing center).

The p.t.a. has also been used to assist with swallowing in infants. The loop in these cases was 0.7 mm and a dental plate was made to fit the baby's upper jaw. It is to be worn all the time until swallowing improves.

Exeter Lip Sensor (figure 16)

The Exeter Lip Sensor is a device that consists of a lip electrode connected to an electronic control unit. The device hooks onto the lower lip and has a wire lip clasp. The center lip electrode is fitted so that the upper lip contacts the electrode when the lips are closed and so completes an electrical circuit. When the lip seal is broken a continuous beep is activated. More recent models of the lip sensor emit a light when the lips are closed and a music or voice tape to play when lip closure is achieved. The lip sensor was developed as a lip seal reminder to assist clients in improving saliva control, nasal breathing, and the production of bilabial consonants.

Prognosis is affected by the following features:

- nasal passages must be clear to enable nasal breathing to occur
- the person should be able to produce a voluntary swallow
- the person has the ability to achieve comfortable lip closure
- the person must be able to tolerate wearing the device for at least 15 to 20 minutes

A study by Callinan, Snelleman, and Vincent (1986) found an increase in lip seal in the two subjects using the Exeter Lip Sensor. However, the evidence for the retention of this skill was inconclusive.

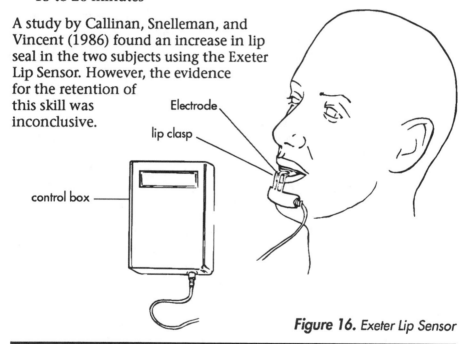

Figure 16. Exeter Lip Sensor

Stimulatory Plates (figure 17)

The use of these appliances was based on the work of Castillo-Morales with "Orofacial Regulation Therapy," initially developed in Argentina in the 1970s.

Fisher-Brandies, Avalle, and Limbrock (1987) investigated the effects of fitting a stimulatory plate on 71 children with cerebral palsy presenting with oral-facial difficulties. The fitting of stimulatory plates was undertaken concurrently with an exercise program based on physiotherapy and speech therapy.

The appliance consists of a metal "stimulator" on a removable orthodontic plate. The design of the stimulator varies with the type of cerebral palsy. For example, some subjects were fitted with a stimulator placed palatally for the tongue and some vestibularly for the upper lip. The plates were intended to inhibit abnormal tongue movement and to facilitate normal movement. They were worn for several hours a day.

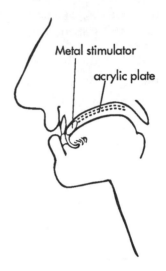

Metal stimulator

acrylic plate

Oral-facial functions were evaluated before and after treatment. Improvements were reported in spontaneous tongue position, drooling, speech development, and coordination of tongue movements in at least 50 percent of the children studied. To attribute this improvement

Figure 17. Stimulatory plate

to the fitting of stimulatorydevices alone was not possible. However, the authors claimed that clinical experience suggested that the changes noted would not have occurred without the use of the device.

Later studies have included similar therapy with children with Down syndrome where significant reduction of oral hypotonic symptoms was claimed.

The Monoblock Appliance

The monoblock appliance, a modified oral shield, was reported to significantly increase nasal breathing and improve tongue position and lip closure in children with cerebral palsy. This was achieved by wearing the appliance to modify malocclusion, over a period of up to two years. Decreased drooling, measured by frequency of wiping, was reported to occur in seven out of nine cases studied. Cooperation of both child and family, together with strict case selection guidelines, was felt to be important to success.

Medications Used in the Control of Oro-Pharyngeal Secretions
(Susan Mathers/Dinah Reddinhough/Amanda Scott)

Excess Secretions and Drooling

Impaired spontaneous swallowing of saliva, poor lip control, or jaw muscle weakness can all result in pooling of oral secretions and potential drooling, especially at mealtimes. Drug treatment is aimed at reducing the flow of saliva by blocking the nerves that are affected by chewing, taste, or emotional stimuli (figure 18).

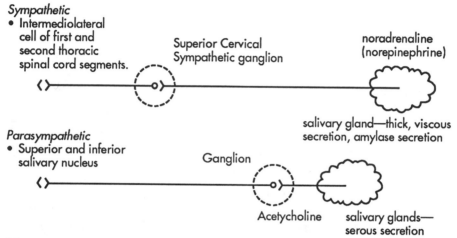

Figure 18. Model of neural mediation of saliva production

Drugs that Reduce Saliva Production

Anticholinergic agents:
- Propantheline Bromide
- Hyoscine (scopolamine)
- Glycopyrronium
- Atropine sulphate
- Benzhexol (Artane)
- Tricyclic antidepressants, Imipramine (Tofranil), Amitriptyline (Tryptanol).

The most commonly used medications have anticholinergic properties that block the parasympathetic innervation of the salivary glands. The parasympathetic nerves regulate the secretion of the fluid component of saliva and therefore anticholinergic drugs primarily reduce the volume of saliva produced and have a lesser effect on the secretion of salivary proteins.

These medications are usually given orally but can be administered by using a transdermal patch (for example, scopoderm [TTS]).

Sympathomimetic drugs/antihistamines:

- Ephredrine
- Pseudoephredrine
- Antihistamines

These drugs are usually found in combination in proprietary decongestant medications for colds and hay fever. As well as blocking immune-mediated secretion from mucous membranes, antihistamines also produce mucosal drying via anticholinergic effects.

Sympathomimetic agents reduce secretions by causing vasoconstriction within the mucous membranes. Since salivary protein secretion occurs primarily in response to sympathetic nerve stimulation, theoretically salivary protein content should increase, resulting in thicker saliva, which may be disadvantageous.

Side effects can include blurred vision, glaucoma, delayed gastric emptying, constipation, urinary retention, flushing, dry skin, tachycardia (palpitations), and confusion.

Some patients find the mouth-drying effect of anticholinergic agents in itself uncomfortable. A reduction in salivary flow rates can result in thicker, more tenacious oro-pharyngeal secretions, which are difficult for patients with oral-pharyngeal weakness to spit out or swallow.

The elderly and patients with dementia or other forms of cortical brain damage may tolerate this type of medication poorly, with increased irritability and confusion.

Patients with glaucoma should not be given anticholinergic medication unless under the strict supervision of an ophthalmologist.

Constipation and urinary retention are troublesome peripheral side effects of anticholinergic medication on the autonomic nervous system. They may require dose limiting, particularly in the elderly or in patients with neurological disease that predisposes them to sphincter disturbance.

Sympathomimetic/antihistamine drugs. Side effects of antihistamines include drowsiness and the anticholinergic side effects described above. Sympathomimetic drugs should be avoided in patients with hypertension or hyperthyroidism, and they are contraindicated in patients taking monoamine oxidase inhibitor drugs for depression.

Adaption and Rebound

A problem that initially was well controlled with medication may return after a period of continuous medication. This occurs when the receptor cells in the salivary glands have adapted to a reduced level of stimulation and become hypersensitive, enabling salivary secretion to return to the pre-medication levels.

A related problem can occur if medication is suddenly stopped. The level of saliva output will have stabilized on the medication; cessation of the medication will lead to a marked increase in output because of induced hypersensitivity of the receptors in the salivary glands. This is known as "the rebound effect." For this reason when medication is to be stopped, it should be tapered off gradually.

Medications that Alter the Consistency of Oral Secretions

Sympathetic nervous system blocking drugs. While parasympathetic nerve stimulation results in increased saliva flow but little salivary protein secretion, animal studies indicate the opposite is achieved with stimulation of the sympathetic innervation of the salivary glands. Sympathetic adrenergic blocking agents, therefore, would not be expected to influence the amount of saliva formed, but may affect its consistency.

It is not clearly understood how cholinergic, adrenergic, and peptidergic neurotransmitters are functionally integrated to modulate saliva production in response to various stimuli.

The use of sympathetic receptor blocking agents is unproven in the treatment of saliva control problems.

Mucolytic agents:
- Citric acid
- Papaya extract
- Acetylcysteine
- Bromhexine

Thick, ropy secretions are difficult to spit out and may obstruct swallowing. Patients with this problem may already have a dry feeling in the mouth and their symptoms are often made worse by the "drying" agents described above. Mucolytic agents are aimed at breaking down the protein contact of mucoid secretions. Citric acid in fruit juices and proteolytic enzymes such as papaya are good first-line therapy. Mucolytic drugs can be administered by inhalation (acetylcysteine) or orally (bromohexine). They can, however, cause gastric irritation.

Choice of Drug and Initiation of Treatment

The role of the medical practitioner is important in prescribing and altering treatment. The choice of medication will be guided by the clinical assessment of the individual patient, taking into consideration any contraindications to specific drugs as outlined above. The assessment can be made more objective by observing the patient at various times of day. Diurnal variation in saliva control problems can also be reported subjectively by the patient using simple charts (see Assessment of Secretions, page 13).

Medication is not always effective in reducing saliva-related problems, and the dosage required for any individual is quite variable. This must be explained at the commencement of treatment. Side effects should be discussed carefully with individuals and their families.

All drugs should be commenced at the lowest dose, given once or twice daily, and increased gradually until optimum effectiveness or limiting side effects occur. Intelligent timing of doses will allow maximum benefit at problem times (for example, meals, social occasions, bedtime). Unless side effects occur, each drug should be given an adequate trial at what is considered by the prescribing clinician to be a full therapeutic dose before being considered ineffective. The dose schedule attained and reasons for withdrawal of the drug should be well documented in the patient's records to guide future management.

Use of medication in the management of drooling in children. Medication is not usually considered a long-term treatment option. However, it is quite useful in a number of situations.

1. It can be used for short periods as an adjunct to behavioral methods, which may be easier to implement with a drier mouth.

2. Drooling may improve spontaneously in children up to the age of about six to seven years. Medication can be valuable in younger children when drooling causes major difficulty, allowing decisions about surgery to be deferred until later.

3. It can be used to assess the advantages of freedom from drooling before surgery is undertaken.

4. It has a role where drooling is a relatively minor problem. Clients may use medication intermittently in situations where drooling will pose a difficulty for them (for example, social situations). One drug that may be used in this way is benzhexol hydrochloride. It begins to act within one hour, the peak effects last two to three hours, and the duration of action is six to twelve hours.

5. Medication may be used for severe drooling over an extended period where:

   a. there has been a reluctance to undergo surgery, or

   b. surgery is contraindicated (for example, in older clients) or with individuals who have terminal conditions

Suggested Protocols for Implementation of Medication

Comment. Given our poor understanding of the complexity of the neural, humoral, and behavioral effects of saliva production and management, it is not surprising that available pharmacological agents can only imperfectly redress the imbalances that lead to saliva control problems.

Accurate assessment and evaluation of response to treatment, therefore, help ensure the most appropriate application of limited therapeutic options.

Protocol 1. A protocol has been adopted for the use of benzhexol hydrochloride (artane) in young children over the age of three years and for teenagers. The dosage is increased over a six-week period. Drooling measurements are taken before medication and once the maximum dose has been reached.

1. The starting dose of benzhexol hydrochloride is 1 mg twice daily for two weeks.

2. If there is no improvement, the dose is increased to 2 mg twice daily for a further two weeks.

3. The dose may be further increased to a maximum dose of 2 mg three times daily.

Protocol 2. A protocol developed to assess the efficacy of medication prescribed to control oral secretions in adults uses an assessment form (refer to form on page 30). As well as documenting the presence of excessive amounts of saliva, this approach also addresses the consistency of the saliva and the daily pattern of the problem. This information helps guide the selection of medication and the timing of doses.

The individual's perception of the problem is discussed. The team members are taught how to use the form. Agreement is reached on how to interpret and quantify the various parameters to be assessed.

Follow-up assessments, using the same form, allow the person's response to dose increments to be monitored.

The Surgical Management of Drooling (Chris Bennett)

The surgical treatment of drooling has evolved slowly, guided by several important principles. Foremost, the operation should be as physiologically sound as possible (this means with minimal changes to the mouth environment) and with limited damage to tissues and surrounding structures. Within this overriding principle lie the following objectives:

- Complications from the operation should be minimal, particularly early problems with swallowing and infection, and late complications such as scars, fistual formation, cysts, and middle ear infections.

- Operative techniques should be used that are the least invasive.

- Hospitalization should be as brief as possible.

- The procedure should be assessed over a long period to determine permanent improvement and long-term complications.

Surgical Methods

Excision of the salivary gland. The simplest method of reducing saliva production is to remove the salivary glands. There are two major sets of paired glands, submandibular and the parotids, and a minor set, sublinguals (see figure 1, page 2). The easiest glands to remove are the submandibular glands. The parotids have rarely been removed, as a major cranial nerve, the facial nerve, runs nearby and there is a risk of damage to that nerve. The other reason it has been popular to remove submandibular glands is that they are one of the largest producers of saliva (about 65 percent). The sublingual glands, which are located close to the submandibulars, are sometimes also removed. Removal of both submandibular glands significantly reduces drooling, but the result is usually temporary. The drooling problem often recurs in about six months, presumably due to an increase in parotid gland output. The operation leaves significant scars on the neck.

Cutting the nerves of the salivary glands. Ear, nose, and throat surgeons have tackled the problem by severing the nerve input to the major salivary glands. This results in a decreased secretion in response to food, smell, and other stimuli. The operation involves minimal hospitalization, but does mean the loss of taste to half of the tongue. There is also a risk of middle ear infection. The early results are good, although the saliva tends to be a bit thick and stringy. The drooling problem also tends to recur over six to twelve months, presumably due to the nerves growing back and growth of parasympathetic pre-ganglionic nerves from other areas.

Cutting the salivary ducts. A simple method of controlling saliva secretion is to ligate (cut) the salivary ducts coming from the major salivary glands. This procedure is practical only with the parotid gland, as it is enclosed within a fibrous capsule that prevents excessive swelling. The ligation is simple, and post-operative complications minimal (this can even be done under a local anesthetic).

There are some concerns about ligating the parotid ducts. These glands produce saliva when eating and drinking and are very useful in assuring the formation of a bolus. It is not practical to ligate the submandibular duct, as this causes considerable swelling in the floor of the mouth and possible airway obstruction. There is also a risk of salivary cyst formation in the floor of the mouth.

The repositioning of saliva glands. The most recent surgical method used to decrease drooling is to reroute the saliva flow from the mouth to the pharynx by transposing the submandibular ducts to the tonsillar fossa at the back of the tongue (see figure 19). This results in saliva now coming out at the back of the throat, rather than pooling in the front of the mouth. It also results in the saliva being swallowed by the involuntary swallow reflex. The parotid ducts are difficult to separate and cannot be relocated satisfactorily. Attempts to elongate the parotid ducts have been abandoned due to complications. Repositioning the submandibular ducts is the most physiologically sound operation, as saliva continues to be produced and is available for swallowing and the early digestion of food. The procedure involves a two-day hospital stay; long-term complications are mainly due to a change in saliva consistency (it becomes thicker and stringy). Short-term problems involve mainly swelling in the floor of the mouth, and a slow start to oral intake due to a painful mouth and throat.

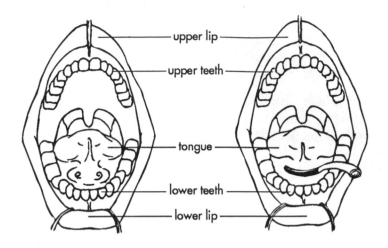

upper lip

upper teeth

tongue

lower teeth

lower lip

Figure 19. Rerouting the submandibular ducts

The Current Surgical Approach in Melbourne, Australia

Our present approach to surgical intervention for drooling is to transpose both submandibular ducts to the tonsillar fossa and to ligate one parotid duct. Patients are all assessed pre-operatively and have usually tried many other methods of saliva control prior to surgery. The hospital stay is two to three days, and both procedures have been chosen to avoid scars completely. Early complications include swelling in the floor of the mouth and cheek, and delayed eating and drinking due to pain. Full recovery usually occurs in one to two weeks. Late complications include thick, stringy saliva, a mucous deposit on the lips, and cyst formation in the floor of the mouth. This last complication is rare (5 percent) but may require a further operation. Any swallowing difficulties have been resolved by adding liquid to the food in the short term. No long-term swallowing problems have occurred. Drooling may also recur after an early improvement, and this usually happens between six and twelve months. Follow-up lasts for two years. Currently a retrospective five-year study is underway.

The *results* of surgery are difficult to interpret. More than 65 patients have had the procedure. The initial improvement appears to decrease with time. Results tend to vary widely, at different times of the day, with different activities, and with stress. The best results are reinforced by behavior management, environmental aids, and intermittent medication. Overall, 30 percent of patients are assessed as very much better by objective testing. Fifty percent of patients are significantly improved, either all the time or for part of the day. Twenty percent of patients have no improvement on testing or subjectively. No patients have been made worse by the surgical treatment. Although it has been reported that dental caries may be more prevalent after surgery, this does not seem to be a significant problem.

In summary, no common pattern can be found to predict the success of surgery. Most patients tend to have a severe problem, and surgery is regarded as a last resort. Those with a milder problem have tended to get better results. The final selection of those patients having surgery usually relates to the severity of the problem at home, at school, and socially.

Chapter 4 COMPENSATORY STRATEGIES FOR DROOLING

Either before or during intervention, in order to improve saliva control, the drooling still has to be dealt with. Sometimes even after all possible interventions a drooling problem will remain.

In these cases, the following strategies are suggested:

Clothing

A very young child can wear a bib to mop up the excess saliva, but this becomes inappropriate as the child grows older. Other ideas you might try are:

1. Using scarves to wear around the neck. (You may need a variety of these in different colors to match various outfits.)

2. Wearing toweling panels for sweatshirts. These can be attached with hook-and-loop fasteners (see figure 20).

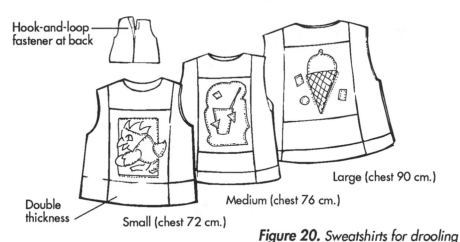

Hook-and-loop fastener at back

Double thickness

Small (chest 72 cm.)

Medium (chest 76 cm.)

Large (chest 90 cm.)

Figure 20. Sweatshirts for drooling

3. Choose sweatshirts with raised motifs (the sweatshirt appears dryer for longer).

4. Terry cloth tops, gathered into a roll neck that fits snugly around the neck.

5. If the child can wipe the chin, try putting sweat bands on the wrist. The chin can be wiped with the wrist rather than the child having to carry a handkerchief.

6. Large lace collars can be interchanged on clothes.

7. Sew an absorbent paper sheet (such as those used as incontinence aids) onto a towel that is worn like a toweling top (figure 21). The sheet absorbs the moisture and does not irritate the skin.

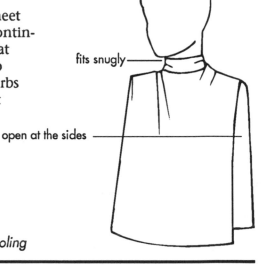

Figure 21. Toweling tops for drooling

Disguising the Odor

Where stale saliva makes clothing smell, try a drop of cologne or deodorizer on the clothes.

Environmental Props

1. Raise the work/school space (by using a slant-board desk, for instance) so that the person does not have to spend long periods with the head down.

2. If the person is in a wheelchair, angle the back of the chair so that the head tips slightly backwards.

3. If the child is hospitalized or in a wheelchair, a goose-neck rod can be attached to the head of the bed or to the wheelchair, with a foam ball on the end. The child can use the foam ball for wiping.

Compensatory Strategies

Dry sticky saliva. Because this may result in a dry mouth or caked saliva on the lips, try:

1. Sucking on fruit lozenges to encourage watery saliva
2. Using lemon glycerine swabs to thin out the saliva in the mouth
3. Spraying the mouth regularly with a water spray
4. Using mouth washes to thin the saliva
5. Using petroleum jelly or lip salve on the lips to keep them from becoming cracked
6. Using artificial saliva (although this does not seem to markedly ease the problem)

Dry mouths. Obviously, drinking will help this condition. Some teas have been found to be most useful (such as lemon tea).

Some teas, however, actually seem to leave the mouth feeling drier (e.g., hibiscus rosehip).

Experiment and try to find the compensatory strategies that most effectively address the specific problems of the client.

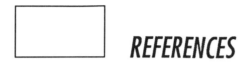

REFERENCES

The Production of Saliva

Andersson, R., E. Arviddson, C. G. Crossner, A. K. Holm, B. Mansson, and H. Grahnen. 1974. The flow rate ph and buffer effect of mixed saliva in children. *Journal of International Association of Dentistry in Children* 5:5-12.

Barylko-Pikielna, N., R. M. Pangborn, and I. L. Shannon. 1968. Effects of cigarette smoking on parotid secretion. *Archives of Environmental Health* 17:731-38.

Baum, B. 1981. Research on aging and oral health: An assessment of current status and future needs. *Special Care in Dentistry* 1(4):145-64.

Birnbaum, D., J. E. Steiner, F. Karmell, and M. Islar. 1974. Visual stimuli and human salivation. *Psychophysiology* 11(3):288-93.

Bogdonoff, M. D., M. Bogdonoff, and S. G. Wolfe. 1961. Studies on salivary function in man. *Journal of Psychosomatic Research* 5:170-79.

Bolwig, T. G., and O. J. Rafaelson. 1972. Salivation in affective disorders. *Psychological Medicine* 2:232-38.

Burgen, A. S. B., and N. G. Emmelin. 1961. *Physiology of the saliva glands* London: Edward Arnold.

Busfield, B. L., H. Weschler, and W. J. Barnum. 1961. Studies of salivation in depression. *Archives of General Psychiatry* 5(11):472-77.

Christensen, C. M., and M. Navazesh. 1984. Anticipatory salivary flow to the sight of different foods. *Appetite* 5:307-15.

Corcoran, D. W. 1964. The relationship between introversion and salivation. *American Journal of Psychology* 77:298-300.

Costa, P. T., H. H. Chauncey, C. O. Rose, and K. K. Kapur. 1980. Relationship of parotid saliva flow rate and composition with personality traits in healthy men. *Oral Surgery* 50:416-22.

Crossner, C. G. 1984. Salivary flow rate in children and adolescents. *Swedish Dental Journal* 8:271-76.

Dawes, C. 1972. Circadian rhythms in human salivary flow rate and composition. *Journal of Physiology* 220:529-45.

Dawes, C., and F. S. Chebib. 1972. The influence of previous stimulation and the day of the week on the concentrations of protein and the main electrolytes in human parotid saliva. *Archives of Oral Biology* 17:1289-1301.

Dawes, C., H. G. Cross, C. G. Baker, and F. S. Chebib. 1978. The influence of gland size on the flow rate and composition of the human parotid gland. *Journal of the Canadian Dental Association* 44(1):21-25.

Dawes, C., and B. Y. Ong. 1973. Circadian rhythms in the flow rate and proportional composition of parotid to whole saliva volume in man. *Archives of Oral Biology* 18:1145-53.

Ekedahl, C., and O. Hallen. 1973. Quantitative measurement of drooling. *Acta Otolaryngology* 75:464-69.

Eysenck, H. J., and S. B. Eysenck. 1967. Salivary response to lemon juice as a measure of introversion. *Perceptual Motor Skills* 24:1047-53.

Fox, P. C., P. F. Ven, B. C. Sonies, J. M. Weiffenbach, and B. J. Baum. 1985. Xerostomia: Evaluation of a symptom with increasing significance. *Journal of American Dental Association* 110:509-15.

Hector, M. P. 1985. The masticatory-salivary reflex. In *Current topics in oral biology,* edited by S. J. W. Lisney and B. Matthews, 320-21. Bristol, U.K.: University of Bristol Press.

Heintze, U., and D. Birkhed. 1984. Influence of a single intake of various test meals on secretion rate, buffer effect and electrolytes of human stimulated whole saliva. *Caries Research* 18:265-68.

Heintze, U., D. Birkhed, and H. Bjorn. 1983. Secretion rate and buffer effects of resting and stimulated whole saliva as a function of age and sex. *Swedish Dental Journal* 7:227-38.

Holmes, J. H. 1964. Changes in salivary flow produced by changes in fluid and electrolyte balance. In *Salivary glands and their secretions,* edited by L. M. Screebny and J. Meyer, 177-95. New York: Macmillan.

Hughes, C, V., B. J. Baum, P. C. Fox, Y. Marmary, C. K. Yeh, and B. C. Sonies. 1987. Oral-pharyngeal dysphagia: A common sequela of salivatory gland dysfunction. *Dysphagia* 1:173-77.

Idowu, A., G. Grase, and S. Handleman. 1986. The effect of age and dentition status on masticatory function in older adults. *Special Care in Dentistry* March-April: 80-83.

Jensen Kjeilin, J. C., P. Brodin, H. Aarss, and T. Berg. 1987. Parotid salivary flow in response to mechanical and gustatory stimulation in man. *Journal of Physiology Scandinavia* 131:169-75.

Kapila, Y. V., W. J. Dodds, J. F. Helm, and W. J. Hogan. 1984. Relationship between swallow rate and salivary flow. *Digestive Diseases and Sciences* 29(6):528-33.

Lagerlüf, F., and C. Dawes. 1984. The volume of saliva in the mouth before and after swallowing. *Journal of Dental Research* 63(5):618-21.

Lourie, R. S. 1943. Rate of the secretion of parotid glands in normal children. *American Journal of Diseases in Children* 65:455-79.

Macgreggor, I. D. M. 1988. Smoking, saliva and salivation. *Journal of Dentistry* 16:14-17.

Muniz, B. R., B. M. Maresca, O. R. Tumilasci, and C. J. Perec. 1983. Effects of an experimental diet on parotid saliva and dental plaque ph in institutionalized children. *Archives of Oral Biology* 28(7):575-81.

Navazesh, M., and C. M. Christensen. 1982. A comparison of whole mouth resting and stimulated salivary measurement procedures. *Journal of Dental Research* 61(10):1158-62.

Palmai, G., and B. Blackwell. 1965. The diurnal pattern of saliva flow in normal and depressed patients. *British Journal of Psychiatry* 111:334-38.

Pangborn, R. M., and I. M. Sharon. 1971. Visual deprivation and parotid response to cigarette smoking. *Physiology Behavior* 6:559-61.

Puskulian, R. 1972. Salivary electrolyte changes during normal menstrual cycle. *Journal of Dental Research* 51:1212-16.

Peck, R. E. 1959. The SHP test—An aid in the detection and measurement of depression. *Archives of General Psychiatry* 1:35-40.

Ramsay, R. W. 1969. Salivary response and introversion-extraversion. *Acta Psychologica* 29:181-87.

Shannon, I. L. 1972. The biochemistry of human saliva in health and disease. In *Proceedings of a symposium on salivary glands and their secretions,* edited by N. H. Rowe. Ann Arbor: University of Michigan School of Dentistry.

Shannon, I. L. 1966. Climatological effects on human parotid gland function. *Archives of Oral Biology* 11:451-53.

Shannon, I. L., and H. H. Chauncey. 1969. Verbal suggestion and parotid flow. *Journal of Oral Medicine.* July: 104-108.

Shannon, I. L., R. P. Feller, and R. P. Suddick. 1971. Light deprivation and parotid flow in the human. *Journal of Dental Research* 51(6):1642-45.

Sreebny, L. M., and G. Broich. 1987. Xerostomia (dry mouth). In *The salivary system,* edited by L. M. Sreebny. Boca Raton, FL: CRC Press, Inc.

Sreebny, L. M., and S. Schwartz. 1986. Reference guide to drugs and dry mouth. *Gerodontology* 5 (1975).

Watnabe, S., and Dawes. 1988. A comparison of the effects of tasting and chewing foods on the flow rate of whole saliva in man. *Archives of Oral Biology* 33(10):761-64.

White, K. D. 1978. Salivation: The significance of imagery and its voluntary control. *Psychophysiology* 15:196-203.

White, K. D. 1975. The significance of individual differences in the control of saliva. Unpublished Ph.D. dissertation, University of Queensland.

Wooley, S. C., and D. W. Wooley. 1974. Salivation to the sight and thought of food. *Psychosomatic Medicine* 35(2):136-42.

Assessment and Measurement

Camp-Bruno, J. A., B. G. Winsberg, A. R. Green-Parsons, and J. P. Abrams. 1989. Efficacy of Benzotropine therapy for drooling. *Developmental Medicine and Child Neurology* 31:309-19.

Dawes, C., and B.Y. Ong. 1973. Circadian rhythms in the flow rate of and proportional composition of parotid to whole saliva volume in man. *Archives of Oral Biology* 18:1145-53.

Gallender, D. 1979. *Eating handicaps.* Springfield, IL: Charles C. Thomas.

Grant, L. 1982. The use of manual vibrator in the speech therapy program of four school-age mentally retarded children. *Journal of Communication Disorders* 15:375-83.

Langley, J. 1987. *Working with swallowing disorders.* Bicester, Oxon: Winslow Press, U.K.

Logemann, J. 1983. *Evaluation and treatment of swallowing disorders.* San Diego, CA: College-Hill Press.

Morris, S. E., and M. D. Klein. 1987. *Pre-feeding Skills.* Tucson, AZ: Therapy Skill Builders.

Sochaniwskyj, A. E., R. M. Koheil, K. Bablich, M. Milner, and D. J. Kenny. 1986. Oral motor functioning frequency of swallowing and drooling in normal children and in children with cerebral palsy. *Archives of Physical Medicine and Rehabilitation* 67:866-73.

Strawbridge, Domaracki, L., and L. A. Sisson. 1990. Decreasing drooling with oral motor stimulation in children with multiple disabilities. *American Journal of Occupational Therapy* 44(8):680-84.

Thomas-Stonell, N., and J. Greenberg. 1988. Three treatment approaches and clinical factors in the reduction of drooling. *Dysphagia* 3:73-78.

Van de Heyning, P. H., J. F. Marquet, and W. L. Creten. 1980. Drooling in children with cerebral palsy. *Acta Oto-Laryngologica Belgica* Tome 34:6.

Approaches to the Management of Drooling

Callinan, F., J. Snelleman, and J. Vincent. 1986. Clinical application of the Exeter Lip Sensor. *Australian Journal of Human Communication Disorders* 14(2):87-93.

Drabman, R., G. Cordua Y Cruz, J. Ross, and S. Lynd. 1979. Suppression of chronic drooling in mentally retarded children and adolescents: Effectiveness of a behavior treatment package. *Behavior Therapy* 10:46-56.

Dunn, K. W., C. E. Cunningham, and J. E. Blackman. 1987. Saliva control and reinforcement in the management of a cerebral palsied adolescent's drooling. *Developmental Medicine and Child Neurology* 29:305-10.

Fisher-Brandies, H., C. Avalle, and G. J. Limbrock. 1987. Therapy of orofacial dysfunctions in cerebral palsy according to Castille-Morales; First results of a new treatment concept. *Journal of Orthodontics* 9:139-43.

Harris, M., and P. F. Dignam. 1980. A non-surgical method of reducing drooling in cerebral palsied children. *Developmental Medicine and Child Neurology* 22:291-99.

Harris, S. P., and A. H. Purdy. 1987. Drooling and its management in cerebral palsy. *Developmental Medicine and Child Neurology* 27:805-14.

Helfrich-Miller, K. R., K. L. Rector, and J. A. Straka. 1986. Dysphagia: Its treatment in the profoundly retarded patient with cerebral palsy. *Archives of Physical Medicine and Rehabilitation* 67:520-25.

Koheil, R., A. Sochaniwskyj, K. Bablich, D. Kenny, and M. Milner. 1987. Biofeedback techniques and behavior modification in the conservative remediation of drooling by children with cerebral palsy. *Developmental Medicine and Child Neurology* 29:19-26.

Rapp, D. 1980. Drool control: Long-term follow-up. *Developmental Medicine and Child Neurology* 22:448-53.

Thomas-Stonell, N., and J. Greenberg. 1988. Three treatment approaches and clinical factors in the reduction of drooling. *Dysphagia* 3:73-78.

Thorbecke, P., and H. Jackson. 1982. Reducing chronic drooling in a retarded female using a multi-treatment package. *Behavior Therapy and Experimental Psychiatry* 13(7):89-93.

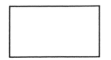 # ADDITIONAL REFERENCES

General

Blasco, P. A., and J. H. Allaine. 1992. Drooling in the developmentally disabled: Management practices and recommendations. *Developmental Medicine and Child Neurology* 34: 849-62.

The Production of Saliva

Brown, C. C. 1970. The parotid puzzle: A review of the literature on human salivation and its applications to psychophysiology. *Psychophysiology* 7:66-85.

Dawes, C., and G. N. Jenkins. 1964. The effects of different stimuli on the composition of saliva in man. *Journal of Physiology* 170:86-100.

Dawes, C., and C. M. Wood. 1973. The contribution of oral motor mucous gland secretions to the volume of whole saliva in man. *Archives of Oral Biology* 18:337-42.

Kerr, C. A. 1961. *The physiological regulation of salivary secretions in man.* London: Pergamon Press.

Kullander, S., and B. Sonesson. 1965. Studies in saliva in menstruating, pregnant and post menopausal women. *Acta endocrinology.* 48:329-31.

Luciano, D. S., A. J. Vander, and J. H. Sherman. 1978. *Human function and structure.* New York: McGraw-Hill.

Norberg, K. A., C. M. Eneroth, and T. Hokfelt. 1970. The significance of the autonomic innervation for the salivary secretion in the human parotid and submandibular glands. *Acta Otolaryngology* 263:193-94.

Sreebny, L. M. 1987. *The salivary system.* Boca Raton, FL: CRC Press, Inc.

White, K. D. 1975. The significance of individual differences in the control of saliva. Unpublished Ph.D. dissertation, University of Queensland.

Assessment and Measurement

Kapila, Y. V., W. J. Dodds, J. F. Helm, and W. J. Hogan. 1984. Relationship between swallow rate and salivary flow. *Digestive Diseases and Sciences* 29(6):528-33.

Lear, C. S. C., J. B. Flannagan, and C. F. A. Moorree. 1965. The frequency of deglutition in man. *Archives Oral Biology* 10:83-99.

Lieblich, S. 1989. Episodic salivation (idiopathic paroxysmal sialorrhea): Description of a new clinical syndrome. *Oral Surgery Oral Medical Oral Pathology* 68(2):159-61.

Spiers, R. L. 1984. Saliva and dental health. *Dental Update* November: 605-12.

Thomas-Stonell, N., and J. Greenberg. 1988. Three treatment approaches and clinical factors in the reduction of drooling. *Dysphagia* 3:73-78.

Measurement of Drooling

Barton, E. J., and J. J. Madsen. 1980. The use of awareness and omission training to control excessive drooling in a severely retarded youth. *Child Behaviour Therapy* 2(1):55-63.

Barton, E. S., E. B. Leigh, and G. Myrvang. 1977. The modification of drooling behavior in the severely retarded spastic patient. *British Journal of Mental Subnormality* 24(47):100-108.

Camp-Bruno, J. A., B. G. Winsberg, A. R. Green-Parsons, and J. P. Abrams. 1989. Efficacy of Benztropine therapy for drooling. *Developmental Medicine and Child Neurology* 31:309-19.

Drabmen, R., Y. Cordua Y Cruz, J. Ross, and S. Lynd. 1979. Suppression of chronic drooling in mentally retarded children and adolescents: Effectiveness of a behavioral treatment package. *Behaviour Therapy* 10:46-56.

Ekedahl, C., and O. Hallen. 1973. Quantitative measurement of drooling. *Acta Otolaryngology* 75:464-69.

Johnson, H. 1990. An exploratory study on drooling using a frequency method of measurement in a naturalistic setting. Unpublished M.S. thesis. La Trobe University, Australia.

Sochaniwiskyj, A. 1982. Drool quantification: Noninvasive technique. *Archives of Physical Medicine and Rehabilitation* 63:605-07.

Approaches to the Management of Drooling

Eating and Drinking Skills

Helfrich-Miller, K. R., K. L. Rector, and J. A. Straka. 1986. Dysphagia: Its treatment in the profoundly retarded patient with cerebral palsy. *Archives of Physical Medicine and Rehabilitation* 67:520-25.

Iammateo, P., C. Trombly, and L. Luecke. 1990. The effect of mouth closure on drooling and speech. *American Journal of Occupational Therapy* 44(8):686-91.

Langley, J. 1987. *Working with swallowing disorders*. Bicester, Oxon, U.K.: Winslow Press.

Logemann, J. A. 1983. Anatomy physiology of normal deglutition. In *Evaluation and treatment of swallowing disorders*. San Diego, CA: College Hill Press.

Morris, S. E., and M. D. Klein. 1987. *Pre-feeding skills*. Tucson, AZ: Therapy Skill Builders.

Sorin, R., S. Somers, W. Austin, and S. Bester. 1988. The influence of video-fluoroscopy on the management of the dysphagic patient. *Dysphagia* 2:127-35.

Starr, S. 1990. Feeding assessment resources management guide. Westmead Hospital, Sydney, Australia.

Oral-Facial Facilitation

Folkins, J. W., and C. Larson. 1978. In search of a tonic vibration reflex in the human lip. *Brain Research* 151:409-12.

Sobsey, R., and F. Orelove. 1984. Neurophysiological facilitation of eating skills in children with severe handicaps. *J.A.S.H.* 9(2):98-110.

Behavior Management

Barton, E. S., E. B. Leigh, and G. Myrvang. 1977. The modification of drooling behaviour in the severely retarded spastic patient. *British Journal of Mental Subnormality* 24(47):100-08.

Burgmayer, S., and Jung. 1983. Hypersalivation in severe mental retardation. *International Journal of Rehabilitation Research* 6:193-97.

Catanese, A. A., and D. A. Sandford. 1984. Head position training through biofeedback: Prosthetic or cure? *Developmental Medicine and Child Neurology* 26:369-74.

Garber, N. 1971. Operant procedures to eliminate drooling behavior in a c.p. adolescent. *Developmental Medicine and Child Neurology* 13:641-43.

Kazdin, A. E. 1989. *Behavior modification in applied settings.* 4th Edition. Pacific Grove, CA: Brooks/Cole.

Ray, S. A., A. C. Bundy, and D. L Nelson. 1983. Decreasing drooling through techniques to facilitate mouth closure. *The American Journal of Occupational Therapy* 37(11):749-53.

Thompson, Iwata B., and H. Poynter. 1979. Operant control of pathological tongue thrust in spastic cerebral palsy. *Journal of Applied Behavior Analysis* 12(3):325-33.

Troft, M. C., and A. D. Maichtlen. 1986. The use of overcorrectness as a means to control drooling. *The American Journal of Occupational Therapy* 40(10):702-704.

Appliances

Bourke, K. J. 1979. "The chewing brush"—Oral physiotherapy. Lecture to 9th Asian Dental Congress. Kuala Lumpur, Malaysia.

Bourke, K. J. How to use the OP device, sometimes known as the "chewing brush" or "munchie." Unpublished article. Maitland, N.S.W., Australia.

Bourke, K. J. 1988. Preventative orthopaedics. Presentation given at the 25th Bicentenary Dental Conference, Sydney, Australia.

Duxbury, J. 1984. Account of a motor neurone disease case and use of palatal training aid. *College of Speech Therapist Bulletin.*

Eastwood, A. W. 1978. The monoblock appliance. *Dental Clinics of North America* 22:739-55.

Haberfellner, H., and B. Rossiwall. 1977. Appliances for treatment of oral sensorimotor disorders. *American Journal of Behavioral Medicine* 56:241-47.

Haberfellner, H., and B. Rossiwall. 1977. Treatment of oral sensorimotor disorders in cerebral palsied children: Preliminary report. *Developmental Medicine and Child Neurology* 19:350-52.

Hoyes, H., and G. J. Limbrock. 1990. Orofacial regulation therapy in children with Down's Syndrome, using the methods and appliances of Castillo-Morales. *Journal of Dentistry for Children* 442-44.

Huskie, C. F., and R. E. Ellis, et al. 1981. The Exeter Lip Sensor in clinical use work in progress. *Bulletin of the College of Speech Therapists* 335:1-5.

Limbrock, G. J., H. Hoyer, and H. Scheying. 1990. Drooling, chewing and swallowing dysfunctions in children with cerebral palsy: Treatment according to Castillo-Morales. *Journal of Dentistry for Children* Nov.-Dec.:445-51.

Oreland, A., J. Heijbel, S. Jagell, and M. Persson. 1989. Oral function in the physically handicapped with or without severe mental retardation. *Journal of Dentistry for Children* 17-25.

Selley, W. G. 1977. Dental help for stroke patients. *British Dental Journal* 143(12):409-12.

Selley, W. G., and J. Boxall. 1986. A new way to treat sucking and swallowing difficulties in babies. *Lancet* 1:1182-84.

Medication Used in the Control of Oro-Pharyngeal Secretions

Bailey, C. M. 1985. Treatment of the drooling child by submandibular duct transposition. *The Journal of Laryngology and Otology* 19:1111-17.

Dworking, J. P., and J. C. Nadal. 1991. Non-surgical treatment of drooling in a patient with closed head injury and severe dysarthria. *Dysphagia* 6:40-49.

Norris, F. H., R. A. Smith, and E. H. Denys. 1985. Motor neurone disease: Toward better care. *British Medical Journal* 291:259-62.

Reddihough, D., H. Johnson, M. Staples, I. Hudson, and H. Exarchos. 1990. Use of benzohexol hydrochloride to control drooling of children with cerebral palsy. *Developmental Medicine and Child Neurology* 32:985-89

Sreebny, L. M., and S. Schwartz. 1986. Reference guide to drugs and dry mouth. *Gerodontology* 5: 1975.

Siegel, L. K., and M. A. Klingbeil. 1991. Control of drooling with transdermal scopalamine in a child with cerebral palsy. *Developmental Medicine and Child Neurology* 33:1013-1014.

Talmay, P. Y., U. Zoehaar, Y. Finklestein, and N. Laurian. 1988. Reduction of salivary flow with scopoderm TTS. *Annals of Otology, Rhinology and Laryngology* 97:128-30.

Thomas, J. (Ed). 1987. *Prescription Products Guide*. 16th Edition. Melbourne: APP Co. Pub.

The Surgical Management of Drooling

Arnrup, K. 1990. Caries prevalence after submandibular duct retroposition in drooling children with neurological disorders. *Pediatric Dentistry* 12(2):98-101.

Brown, A. S. 1985. A team approach to drool control in cerebral palsy. *Annals of Plastic Surgery* 15:5.

Burton, M. J. 1991. The surgical management of drooling. *Developmental Medicine and Child Neurology* 19:514-417.

Cotton, R. T. 1981. The effect of submandibular duct rerouting in the treatment of sialorrhoea in children. *Otolaryngology Head and Neck Surgery* 89:341-353. July to August.

Crysdale, W. S. 1980. The drooling patient: Evaluation and current surgical options. *Laryngoscope* 90:775-83.

Crysdale, W. S. 1982. Submandibular duct relocation for drooling—How to do it. *Journal of Otolaryngology* 11:286-88.

Crysdale, W. S. 1985. The drooling patient: Team evaluation and management. International Journal of Paediatric *Otorhinolarynology* 9:241-48.

Crysdale, W. S. 1989. Management options for the drool patient. *Ear, Nose, and Throat Journal* 68:820-39.

Crysdale, W. S., and A. White. 1989. Submandibular duct relocation: A 10-year experience in 194 patients. *Journal of Otolaryngology Head and Neck Surgery* 101(1):87-92.

Makhani, J. S. (1974). Dribbling of saliva in children with cerebral palsy and its management. *Indian Journal of Paediatrics* 41:272-277.

Wilkie, J. F. 1970. The surgical treatment of drooling. *Plastic and Reconstructive Surgery* 45(6):549-54.

Wilkie, T. F. 1977. The surgical treatment of drooling. *Plastic and Reconstructive Surgery* 59(6):791-97.

Provide assistance with these materials for your clients who have feeding and swallowing disorders. . .

PRE-FEEDING SKILLS
A Comprehensive Resource for Feeding Development
by Suzanne Evans Morris, Ph.D., CCC-SLP, and Marsha Dunn Klein, M.Ed., OTR/L

Here's a problem-solving approach to remediating oral-motor disorders. This resource includes comprehensive information from anatomy and normal development to assessment and treatment. It includes 52 Participation Experiences giving you the opportunity to be an active participant in learning and more than 550 illustrations. **0761674063-YCS**

FEEDING AND SWALLOWING DISORDERS IN INFANCY
Assessment and Management
by Lynn S. Wolf, M.O.T., OTR, and Robin P. Glass, M.S., OTR

This practical resource integrates information in the areas of sucking, swallowing, and breathing to aid in evaluation and treatment of infants ages birth to 1 year. Problem-solving models provide a systematic and logical approach for clinicians working with specialized infant feeding disorders. You'll have case studies, reference lists, and discussions of strengths and weaknesses of different approaches. **0761641904-YTS**

ORAL-MOTOR/FEEDING RATING SCALE
by Judy Michels Jelm, M.S., CCC-SLP

This adaptive resource helps you screen and categorize the many varieties of oral-motor movements and note specific patterns as your client eats a typical meal. Ideal for initial observations of skill levels, re-evaluating previously observed skills, or as a framework for developing your own therapy plan. The clear, concise format can be used in a variety of settings in less than an hour! **0761647023-YTS**

SWALLOWING DISORDERS (Revised)
What Families Should Know
by Tom Rader, M.S., CCC-SLP, and Barbara Rende, M.S., CCC-SLP

These easy-to-follow booklets are useful resources for parents, families, and caregivers in home programming, workshops, and inservice training. Each booklet offers a case history, stages and symptoms of swallowing disorders, a glossary, and professional resources list. Sold in sets of 10. **076163004X-YCS**

WORKING WITH SWALLOWING DISORDERS
A Multidisciplinary Approach
by Jill C. Thresher, M.A., CCC-SLP, and Ellis A. Kehoe, M.Ed., OTR/L

Using an integrated team-based approach, you can ensure consistent treatment of adults who have neurogenic oral-pharyngeal dysphagia as a result of stroke, head injury, or progressive neurological diseases. This manual provides an outline for starting your multidisciplinary team. You'll be able to provide step-by-step guidelines for stages of management including referral, screening, assessment, treatment, and discharge. Reproducible forms assist you in every phase. **0761678077-YCS**

SWALLOWING INSTRUCTION SHEETS AND STICKERS
by Margaret Keck Dickey, M.A., CCC-SLP, and Sue Clawson Wilkinson, M.A., CCC-SLP

Use these easy-to-see stickers and sheets to show caregivers the correct swallowing instructions to follow. Each color-coded 25-sheet pad represents a different level of swallowing ability. The 1½" x 1¼" stickers show positioning techniques and specifics on food and liquids. They're versatile so you can meet the needs of all your clients with dysphagia—mix and match to create individualized programs. **0761676805-YCS**

MANAGING DYSPHAGIA
An Instructional Guide for the Client and Family
by Brad Hutchins, M.A., CCC-SLP

Promote home carryover of dysphagia goals, treatment, and compensatory techniques with this video and informational workbooks. Motivate clients and families to participate fully in the rehabilitation process, while you save valuable explanation time! Using a single-family approach, total administration time takes only 30 minutes. **0761678034-YCS**

MAROON SPOONS

You're going to want to order in quantities for home carryover. The narrow, shallow bowl allows food to slide off easily and the durable plastic construction stands up against reflex biting. Dishwasher safe, too!

Small (1" bowl), 0761641564-YTS (set of 25)
Large (1¼" bowl), 0761641572-YTS (set of 25)

FLEXI CUPS

Flexi Cups help you promote proper cup drinking. Choose from 1-oz., 2-oz., and 7-oz. flexible dishwasher-safe cups. The generously cut-out rim makes this cup an invaluable feeding tool! The flexible material allows you to control the shape of the cup by gently squeezing the sides.

0761642676-YTS (1 oz./pink) (set of 5)
0761647066-YTS (2 oz./blue) (set of 5)
0761642684-YTS (7 oz./lime green) (set of 5)

For current prices on these practical resources, please call 1-800-228-0752.

Spend more time with your clients, less time record-keeping with these helpful professional resources . . .

REPORT WRITING FOR SPEECH-LANGUAGE PATHOLOGISTS

by Grace F. Middleton, Ed.D., CCC-SLP, Mary H. Pannbacker, Ph.D., CCC-SLP, Gay T. Vekovius, M.S., CCC-A, Valerie Puett, M.S., CCC-SLP, and Kathryn L. Sanders, M.S., CCC-SLP

This excellent tool provides you with an organized means of teaching report writing in small steps. Using a series of short assignments, clinicians and soon-to-be clinicians learn to include necessary information in reports such as ethical considerations and technical aspects. Handle various types of reports, organize reports appropriately, complete reports in a timely fashion, and write quality comprehensive reports. **0761677976-YCS**

PLANNING INDIVIDUALIZED SPEECH AND LANGUAGE INTERVENTION PROGRAMS
Objectives for Infants, Children, and Adolescents (Revised)
by Nickola Wolf Nelson, Ph.D., CCC-SLP

This 620-page guide helps you save planning time and features an in-depth discussion of the goal area, complete with references and other useful information for planning remediation. Plus, it provides the latest information about effective programming. You'll have 46 sets of objectives organized into 14 goal areas including Prespeech, Early Language, Written Language, Hearing Impairment, and Fluency. **0761622756-YCS**

DESK REFERENCE OF ASSESSMENTS IN SPEECH-LANGUAGE

by Lonnie G. Harris, Ph.D., CCC-SLP, and Ivy Skaife Shelton, M.S., CCC-SLP

Keep on top of the latest developments in assessments! You'll have detailed reviews of 90 commercially available testing instruments for your clients of all ages. Reviews for each instrument include general information, normative data, procedures, and objective evaluations. **0761671668-YCS**

Here's a functional resource for your clients with head injury . . .

STEP-BY-STEP MEALS
For People with Cognitive Challenges
by Nancy Rose Nightingale, M.P.H., RN, and Jennifer Lyn Nightingale

Take your clients who have impaired cognition through all the steps of meal planning and preparation with this delightful book. There are 18 entire meals—each has a comprehensive activity analysis promoting functional independence for your clients. You'll save time in the clinic and during home carryover programs because you no longer have to convert recipes—the step-by-step process is already done for you! **0761642870-YTS**

ORDER FORM

Ship to:

Institution: _____

Name: _____

Occupation/Dept: _____

Address: _____

City: _____ State: _____ Zip: _____

Please check here if this is a permanent address change. ☐

Telephone No._____ ☐ work ☐ home

Payment Options:

☐ Bill me. ☐ My check is enclosed. ☐ My purchase order is enclosed. P.O. # _____

☐ Charge to my credit card: ☐ VISA ☐ MasterCard ☐ American Express

Card No. ☐☐☐☐☐☐☐☐☐☐☐☐☐☐☐☐☐☐

Expiration Date: Month _____ Year _____

Signature _____

Qty.	Cat. #	Title	Amount

Prices are in U.S. dollars. Payment must be made in U.S. funds only.

- If your account is not currently listed as "tax exempt," applicable destination charges will be added to your invoice.
- Orders are shipped by United Parcel Service (UPS) unless otherwise requested. If another delivery service is required, please specify.
- For regular delivery service, your order will be charged 5% handling plus actual shipping charges.
- We occasionally backorder items temporarily out of stock. If you do not accept backorders, please tell us on your purchase order or on this form.

Money-Back Guarantee

You'll have up to 90 days of risk-free evaluation of the products your ordered. If you're not completely satisfied with any product, we'll pick it up within the 90 days and refund the full purchase price! **No questions asked!**

For Phone Orders

Call 1-800-228-0752. Please have your credit card and/or institutional purchase order information ready. Monday-Friday 7am-7pm Central Time.
1-800-723-1318 TDD FAX 1-800-232-1223

Send your order to:

Communication Skill Builders

a division of The Psychological Corporation
555 Academic Court / San Antonio, Texas 78204-2498